What Others Say About This Book

"For the first time in my life my hair and I are friends."
Thank you for writing this book! At first I was reticent and realized that I was resisting thinking about hair as an issue. My opinion, based on my own experience, is that hair for women of African descent is an issue of self esteem and that at its real foundation, hair is an issue of safety and survival…for the first time in my life my hair and I are friends. It is wash and go. My scalp is healthy. I am trying to get the rest of my life as focused and hassle free.
—Ava H. Stanley, MD – Somerset, NJ

"This book has given me a wake up call"
All the books I have read so far have dealt with the maintenance of hair; never has anyone addressed the issue of why so many of us consistently abuse ourselves chasing an impossible dream. I will never know if my hair loss could have been prevented, but I do know this book has given me a wake-up call. At 40 something, I have just begun my journey down the road of recovery… your book has helped me to gain the inner peace I longed for. Thank you again.
—Jacqueline Ricks – Washingtonville, NY

"…This book is so true…"
What is being stated in this book is so true but we don't realize it. I used to make fun of young Black women who wore their hair natural…now I can say that my mother wears natural hair (locks) and because of her wearing the natural look, it makes me look more positively at other women who wear the same look.
—Isiah Jones – Asbury Park, NJ

"What a great and important book"
I just wanted to take the time to drop you a line to let you know what a great and important book… you have written. It really helped me stay focused in my quest to grow a healthy head of natural hair… Thanks to your book, you can add me to the list of sisters who will never chemically straighten my hair again! Your book really tells the history of our hair and

it is every bit unique and glorious …Thank you for such an informative book.

—Deidra W. Gray - Copperas Cove, TX

"This book has confirmed some of my worries…"

This book has confirmed some of my worries that I have chosen to ignore for the sake of vanity. It has made me take a hard and close look at what I am doing to my hair and scalp. —Barbara Lewis – Teaneck, NJ

"Instills pride in having Black hair"

This book not only gives the history of present beliefs about Black hair but also promotes and instills pride in having Black hair, being proud of oneself and heritage and wearing black hair naturally and proudly.

—Sharon Stafford - St. Clair Shores, MI

"After reading this book, I found myself staring at everyone…"

I personally, being white, have not given much thought to the matter of African hair…but it was obvious to me that the material contained in this informative book was well researched. Also evident, is the compassion of the authors towards the healing of such a sensitive subject. It is extremely sad to me that all these years removed from the enslavement period African people must suffer from its ramifications, right down to the hair follicle! After reading this book, I found myself staring at everyone carefully; studying their hair.

—Marie A. Leiggi-Bell – Trenton, NJ

"This book has inspired me."

I really enjoyed this book. I have already recommended it to several people… The book was extremely informative and broadened my mind on this subject. It has also helped me understand… how the deeply rooted psychological effects of slavery continued to affect us today. This book has inspired me.

—Jeffery Brutus – East Orange, NJ

Media Raves About This Book and The Authors

Through text, photographs, and drawings, Black Folk's Hair argues—with an insistence that is bound to spark anger in some readers...
—Star-Ledger Newspaper

The book, which attempts to unravel the reason behind the "mutilation" of black hair, is invigorating and thought provoking...the very thing we need in black communities...May ruffle some feathers.
—The Voice Newspaper

A Hair-Straightening Experience! Research on 'black folks hair' yields insight into African-American style.
—The Focus Newspaper

The Kenyattas have made some interesting discoveries on the hair-straightening subject.
—The Courier News

Black Folk's Hair
Secrets, Shame & Liberation
Revisited

Kamau & Janice Kenyatta

Songhai Publications
Albrightsville, PA

Black Folk's Hair: Secret, Shame & Liberation - Revisited

Library of Congress Control Number:2019915416

ISBN 0-9650653-3-2

Printed in the United States of America

Published by:
Songhai Publications
105 Reynolds Road
Albrightsville, PA 18210

Cover photo by Simon Wakaba - unsplahed.com
This image is from Unsplash and was published prior to 5 June 2017 under the Creative Commons CC0 1.0 Universal Public Domain Dedication

Dedicated to Samiya, Kamauri, Mya, Nyla and future generations.

Contents

x

Introduction

We are fully aware that the subject matter of this book is one that is sensitive for Black people in general and Black women in particular and that it touches a tender and age-old wound. With this in mind, note that we view this work as an effort to heal this wound and not as an attempt to administer unnecessary pain. We do not, however, apologize for the pain that some will encounter as they progress through the book. We know that is a necessary part of the healing process because it dares to address one of the deep wounds that remain unattended from the enslavement and the colonization of African people.

Although it addresses an external feature of our African-ness, it really speaks to a deeper psychological malady. And while we specifically direct the contents of this book toward Black women, our aim is not to bash these women. Neither is it our intention to overlook those Black men who engage in the practice of straightening their hair or those who ridicule Black women who wear natural styles. The latter group remains part of the ongoing problem. Nevertheless, our experience indicates and evidence shows that Black women straighten their hair in far greater numbers than Black men. That cannot be logically or intelligently contested.

Responses To The Book

Since writing the first edition of this book under the initial title *Black Folk's Hair: Secrets, Shame & Liberation*, a few things have happened that are worthy of mention. First, the response to the book was received and welcomed in places we had not intended nor anticipated.

For example, the positive responses and reactions of white women to the book was completely unforeseen. But even more shocking is the fact that many of them bought additional copies to give as gifts to their "Black girlfriends." Along those same lines we found that many white women who have children by Black men have bought the book in great numbers in order to better understand the hair of their children from those unions. This was not an intended market for the book but one that, nonetheless, has been beneficial to many and one that we see as a necessary part of the discussion.

Secondly, the rapidity with which news of the book spread into other parts of the world was a welcomed surprise. Two specific occasions regarding this come to mind. On one occasion, we received a phone call from the Netherlands from Black women seeking copies of the book and inviting us to speak at a conference there. On another occasion, we received orders for copies of the book from Germany that totally floored us.

Thirdly, the impact the book has had on women has been tremendous. Some have read the book and immediately decided to go natural. Others have gone natural after much debate, inner turmoil and soul searching. For example, several of my former students who argued with me (Kamau) as to why they would never wear natural hair have come back a few months or a few years later wearing natural hairstyles. Others have taken a defiant stance claiming they wouldn't be caught dead with so-called "nappy" hair. Still there are those who have had to change to natural styles due to health reasons.

In all the cases that we've witnessed, where women have gone natural, no one has ever expressed any remorse or regret about their decision. None of them became ugly or uglier (as some thought they would) because they had previously accepted the notion that they would and could not be beautiful with their natural hair. To our knowledge and experience they are all happy and delighted with their newfound beauty. There is no power like the power of being yourself—none.

Another unexpected surprise has come from Black men who have purchased the book to give to the women in their lives—mothers, sisters, wives, nieces, cousins and girlfriends. It is also worth mentioning that our predictions in 1996 that more women would begin to wear natural hairstyles has been proven correct. We also predicted that there would be an increase in the number of natural hair salons around the country and that, too is proving to be correct.

Why We Changed The Title

The title of the book has been changed back to the original first edition title. We thought that changing the title to *The Truth About Hairstyles: The Whole Story Revealed,* would have a broader appeal and help with the sales of the book. That has proven to be untrue. And so, we have returned the book to its original title. We consider this work as part of the overall Afrocentric project, which endeavors to restore, reconstruct, and return African people to themselves.

What You Will Find In The Book

In Chapter 1 we discuss the unique quality and beauty of African hair, while also broaching the subject of enslavement's psychological implications and impact on Black folk's hair. Chapter 2 looks at the origins of the present attitudes African people have regarding their hair as a result of the European enslavement of African people.

Chapter 3 discusses the ways in which we speak of our hair and the aesthetic value(s) we have internalized. We also discuss the different techniques used to straighten Black hair.

In Chapter 4 we provide the results of surveys we conducted among women who straighten their hair and among those who wear their hair natural. In addition, this chapter highlights some of the current practices evidenced in the shift toward natural hairstyles by more Black women.

Chapter 5 examines the impact chemicals may have on the health of those who receive relaxers and those who apply relaxers. In the final chapter, we look at the economic factors associated with the Black hair care industry and provide a list of hair products by Black-owned companies and White-owned companies.

Throughout the book we have used the words Black and African interchangeably, and we have intentionally used the uppercase lettering for Black.

Although we have used African Americans for most of our examples, this book and its subject matter is not only addressing that group of Africans. The practice of straightening African hair is found among practically all African groups whether they reside in the Americas, the Caribbean, or on the continent of Africa. This work, therefore, is directed toward African people wherever they may be found.

The Purpose of This Book

It is our hope that this work will create an atmosphere where the subject of Black hair might be openly discussed and given more careful and reflective thought. We hope that such an atmosphere might create a renewed appreciation and love for our natural hair. We also hope that this work will (1) motivate and inspire sisters (and brothers) to wear their natural hair proudly, (2) help Black men become supportive of women who go natural, and (3) challenge the system that penalizes us for being our true selves and true to ourselves.

We must learn to love our hair just as it is and we must totally accept ourselves, and those like us. If we cannot accept ourselves entirely, it may be because we do not really love ourselves, or our people as we may profess, and thus we run the risk of becoming false, fake, and phony. African people are a great people, but as long as we hate any part of ourselves, we are doomed to the exile reserved only for those who fail to see their own greatness as humans.

Kamau Kenyatta
Janice Kenyatta

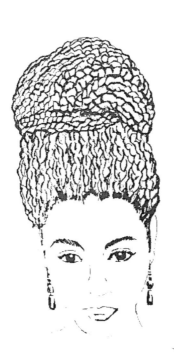

Somebody tell me, what they tryin' to hide? 'Cause what you're looking for it's been here with you all the time.
— Peter Tosh —

You running and you running and you running away...You running and you running and you running away...But you can't run away from yourself.
— Bob Marley —

Chapter 1

Black Hair: The Best Kept Secret

Several years ago my husband came home one evening from an African American history and cultural class and made a suggestion that would result in a knockdown, drag out, verbal fight that has since changed my way of life. At the time, it seemed like the most outrageous and absurd suggestion he had ever presented to me. I could not believe that he was serious about what he was asking. Deep down inside, however, he had struck a cord that within myself I knew would not go away. What did he suggest? He suggested I stop relaxing my hair and wear it natural. Until then I had never given any serious thought concerning why I relaxed my hair.

In the early 1970s I wore an Afro with pride because that was the style of the times and also an expression of the "Black-is-Beautiful era." Since that era, I returned, like so many others from that period, to relaxing my hair. My husband's question to me was, *"Janice, why do you straighten your hair?"* Of course, I gave him the usual excuses of straight hair being easier to manage, natural hair not fitting my face, my employer reacting negatively, and the negative reactions of my family and friends. In retrospect, I had no substantial satisfactory answers to give him. It did not occur to me that I could be just as beautiful with my natural hair as I thought I was with my artificially straightened hair and with less effort.

A year after Kamau posed that earth-shattering question (and for many women of African descent, it was and continues to be an *"earth-shattering question"*) I made the conscious and deliberate decision to go natural. Why? Because I came to the realization that:

(1) Black folk's hair is beautiful in its natural state. It's not ugly.

(2) given an understanding of the historical reality of how and why Black people straighten their hair, I could no longer engage in such an obvious denial of my God-given attribute.

To begin the process of eliminating my artificially straightened hair, I first moved to braids (extensions) in order to allow my natural hair to grow and flourish. I was amazed with the ease and manageability of this hairstyle. In addition, when I took the braids out after a few months, I discovered that I had grown a head full of healthy natural hair. Inspired by this, and raising two infant daughters, I decided to try a natural short cut, which I wore for a little over a year. By this time, I had come to love and admire my natural hair to the extent that I began to realistically consider wearing locks. This, for me, was an easy and natural transition. Although locks may not be for everyone, and we are not advocating that they are, during this phase of my life, I discovered that no other style compared with the ease of manageability, versatility, and elegance of this hairstyle.

I wore locks for 18 consecutive years while cutting them periodically to obtain a shorter, sassy Bob type hairstyle. Sometimes I would let them grow very long all the way down my back. Ultimately, after 18 years, I decided to cut my locks off completely, and since that time, I continue to rock short, tapered natural cuts at varying lengths. The convenience and manageability of this look fits well into my active lifestyle!

I might add that during those 18 years of wearing locks and later wearing the short natural cuts, I was employed as a teacher, high school administrator and a college administrator. Wearing my hair natural was not a factor of employment.

Reflecting upon my previous thinking about natural hair, I now understand that I operated from a lack of information about African hair. Unfortunately, many Black women and men still think the way I once thought. I realize that the majority of them lack the necessary information, which was instrumental in helping me make the transition from straightened hair to natural hair. I owe this awakening to my husband who first challenged, encouraged, enlightened, and supported me in this endeavor. We have co-written this book in order to educate, inform, challenge and inspire Black women and men to love their hair.

Why This Book?

Imagine walking into any assembly of Black people e.g., church, school, college, shopping mall, street corner, bar, dance hall etc., in almost any part of the world. In that instance, we would see the majority of Black women wearing their hair artificially straightened in such styles involving relaxers, hot-combs, bone straight weaves and wigs. They have become the rule. Despite the promising progress we have seen toward the acceptance of natural hair, Black women who wear their hair in naturals, i.e. short cuts, braids, and locks are primarily considered as the exception to the rule when we look at the total picture. Black men, on the other hand, as a rule wear their hair natural, and those few who do straighten it are the exception.

Rarely does anyone think to ask why do the majority of Black women *still* straighten their hair. In your own experience, how many times have you asked or heard someone ask a Black woman, *"Why do you straighten your hair?"* We would venture to gamble our future earnings that less than 1% of Black people ever pose the question regarding this pervasive and accepted practice, and when all is said and done, we would win the bet. As an exercise, count the number of Black women you see wearing natural styles, and compare it with the number you see wearing artificially straightened hair. The results will be revealing. But that's not all because...

Another perplexing peculiarity occurs when we hear Blacks (women specifically) assert that *"we should love ourselves and be proud of ourselves."*

We've all heard this statement before or one similar. How was the sister wearing her hair? The issue of equating self-love with wearing our natural hair has not been a concern for most Black people. In fact, many naively think it's irrelevant and there are bigger and more pressing issues facing Black people. Yet, artificially straightened hair is such an obvious denial of self-love, but one that goes unnoticed and unquestioned. What do these people mean when they say we should love ourselves and be proud of ourselves? **_Do they mean we should love all of ourselves except our hair?_** Is our hair somehow separate from the rest of our anatomy and not deserving of just as much love? Some black women will justify this fact, by commenting that they have great self-esteem and that the way they choose to wear their hair has nothing to do with self-esteem. Our studies and observations point to a direct correlation between the way a woman chooses to wear her hair and her self-esteem. This fact applies to White women as well.

African hair is unique. It has no equal on the planet, and the truth is Black people do not like it. This is because we were systematically taught to hate our own hair, while at the same time we were taught to love and admire the hair of White people — straight hair. This continues to be a hard and bitter pill for our people to swallow.

The hatred is so deep that most of us are not even consciously aware that we hate our hair. But the hatred manifests itself not only in what we do to it but more importantly by the way we speak of it — always in negative and derogative terms: "nappy this, knotty that, peasy headed so and so," etc. This indicates a deep level of hatred for the African's hair. Until recently, rarely, if ever, did we hear anyone speaking of it in endearing or fond terms. On the other hand, what we do to it indicates our attempts to hide it, cover it up, or disguise it so no one will know who we really are. It is but one more perennial attempt to be more like White people whom we believe are superior by virtue of our experience and education.

In attempting to straighten our hair, we indirectly inform Whites that they are correct. Our actions say that they are superior and that we will do anything and everything to be like them or as near like them as possible. This is absurd and insane! Despite the protests we hear to the contrary, actions do speak louder than words.

Almost every other group or race of people on the planet has some type of straight hair except the majority of African people. But since Europeans have colonized and controlled the world, they have, for the past 500 years, bombarded the world with the idea and the image of themselves as the most beautiful and the most glorious people of all the peoples of the earth. A large part of that bombardment is the untruth that straight hair is the hair that everyone should have if they are to be considered beautiful and acceptable. No other people have been more susceptible to this lie than African peoples. This includes those in North America, South America, the Caribbean, Europe and on the continent of Africa.

We have been attempting to straighten our hair for so long now that it is accepted as normal. The truth is this is not normal behavior. Straight hair is not the most beautiful hair, nor the only beautiful hair; it is not the easiest hair to manage; it is not the standard of beauty for people who do not have it. We are operating in the arena of self-deception if we accept such a conclusion as the truth. If and when we do, we in effect say that the CREATOR did not have infinite wisdom in giving us the type of hair we have. We say by our words and more importantly our actions that the CREATOR made a mistake or an error, and we must somehow "improve" upon it. Thus, all attempts at such alterations deny the wisdom of the Divine.

Can You Imagine This?

Imagine walking into a room filled with White women wearing Afro wigs, braids, or locks. What would you think? Most people, if they were honest, would wonder why are they trying to be like Blacks? Most would also acknowledge that the Whites are in fact imitating Black people. We would find their behavior strange and unusual to say the least. The same dynamics do not apply, however, when the equivalent scenario is presented in regard to Black women. For example, imagine you walked into the same room as before but now it consists of a room full of Black women wearing their hair artificially straightened, straight weaves sown/glued to their scalp or straight haired wigs. You/We would not think that it was strange or unusual. We would not even question why Black women are engaging in such a practice. That scenario is in fact accepted as normal.

What is it that would allow us to readily notice as peculiar or abnormal a room full of White women attempting to make their hair like Blacks, but does not allow us to notice the same peculiarity or abnormality when we walk into a room full of Black women attempting to wear their hair straight like Whites? To add insult to injury, Black women who proudly wear short natural styles and locks are often asked by other Black brothers and sisters why they wear their hair "like that?" The natural styles are perceived as somehow peculiar or abnormal.

Returning to our scenario, what if one of those White women, wearing her hair like Blacks, said to an audience of Whites on TV, in church, or at a school, *"You should love yourselves and be proud of yourselves."* Would you not see a gross contradiction between her words and her actions? Would you not cringe at the obvious conflicting message being sent, especially to young white children? Of course you would. But Black women (and some Black men) do this all the time all over creation and we never even bat an eye. We applaud the obvious contradiction, and we never question the practice.

These double messages are sent to Black youth from an early age. In fact, those same double messages were sent to Black adults when they were children and thus helps to explain, in part, why we can see the abnormality in others, but not see the same abnormality in ourselves. What in reality has been created is a case of the blind leading the blind.

Do You Know Why We Have Hair?

According to the authors of *The Journey of the Songhai People*, protection of the brain is the foremost reason for hair on the head. When we consider the significance of the brain to life and reality, this assertion is quite credible. We may lose an arm, a leg, or a hand and still function at peak levels because the brain is intact. We may become paralyzed, losing the use of over 50% of our body and still function at a very high level of achievement. In fact, many people who are confined to wheelchairs are more resourceful and accomplish more than some people who have full use of their body faculties. This is because their brain has not been affected or damaged to the extent that their mental growth is impeded. On the other hand, if the brain is slightly damaged, all of life, as one knows it is altered, in some cases, forever.

The human brain is the central control of our consciousness. It controls every single function we endeavor from the smallest detail to the most exacting task. It is also the quintessential example of evolution in humanity. As such, it represents the sum total of one's conscious identity. One may have false teeth, false eyelashes, false eyes, or one's heart, liver, or kidney may be replaced, but if one were to cut out a minute section of the brain, one's conscious identity would be forever altered or lost.

Understanding the importance of the human brain, nature provided it the maximum protection. It is housed first in a protective sac, floating in a protective liquid to absorb jarring, covered with a bony shield called a skull. The skull is covered with a rubbery mesh of tissues called the scalp, and the scalp is covered with hair. No other part of the human anatomy is so well protected, not even the heart! [1]

There is some difference of opinion concerning whether Black hair is dead or alive. For example, author Nekena Evans (and many others) posits that it is alive. She observes that *"we can say with assurance that hair is alive, particularly hair that is coiled."*[2] Her conclusion is that because it responds to atmospheric conditions such as the weather and seasons and requires the same basic cosmic food of the universe as any other living entity such as air, sunshine, moisture, and earth it must, therefore, be alive. Others, however, assert that it is dead since hair does not have the ability to reproduce itself. While each side makes worthy points for consideration, some type of scientific analysis would best settle the debate.

What Evans does point out, with a degree of certainty, is that "hair also acts as a natural biofeedback system, responding to stress and internal dietary states." [3]

Spiritually, our hair houses our ancient race/cultural memory and our ancestral connections. It connects us to our heritage and roots in the most intimate of ways, and it provides us with a mechanism of "storing and transmitting electromagnetic energy" that functions much like antennae. Just as the environment influences plants (atmospheric conditions, touch, speech, diet, etc.) so is the African hair affected, and ultimately these factors eventually impact the entire body. Persons who wear their hair in locks are probably more acutely attuned to these dynamics than others.

Personally speaking, while wearing our locks, we became aware of an acute sensitivity to the spiritual realm or a heightening of what some refer to as the sixth sense or intuition.

Given this understanding of African hair, it is incumbent upon us to consider what happens to us psychologically and spiritually when we apply harsh chemicals, hot combs, heavy oils (grease), and glue to our hair and scalp. In effect, we literally destroy it. *(See Chapter 5 for more)* The optimum solution thereafter, if the damage is not too severe, is to grow a new head of hair less these detrimental impositions. In reality, however, most people who do these things to their hair never give it a chance to recover. Thus, the electromagnetic energy is destroyed, the biofeedback system does not work properly, and we lose the intimate ancestral connections. [4]

What Makes Black Hair Unique?

The authors of *The Journey of the Songhai People* assert that the hair of the African is structured in such a way as to give the maximum external protection to the brain. The hair serves as the first form of defense for the brain. Without getting bogged down in a minute discussion of the hair texture of the African, yet avoiding over-simplification, let us briefly recapitulate their explanation. They observed four things when looking at the hair of the African under a microscope:

1. *As the hair shaft automatically evolves from the follicle, it becomes alive and raises itself from the scalp. This forms a halo to affect a cushion against blows or falls.*
2. *To strengthen the cushion effect, the hair shaft automatically forms waves with spring-like characteristics.*
3. *Each hair shaft grows hooking tendrils on each side, which hooks onto the adjacent hair shaft. This forms a woven halo to protect against penetration of objects, which could*

penetrate the skull and damage the brain. (See illustration)

4. *The shape of the hair shaft is not cylindrical (round), but ribbon or flat shaped. This gives the tendrils the ability to grow into the weaving* affect. [5]

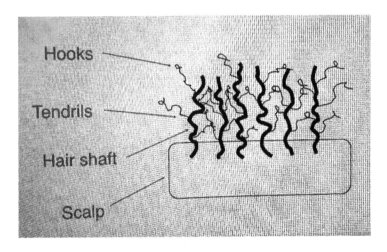

Cross-section of African/Black hair

The tendrils in truly African hair are so strong that when attempts are made to comb this type of hair, the teeth of the comb may break.

Since combing this type of hair with combs designed for straight hair breaks the tendrils, the amount of external protection to the brain is slightly reduced. Therefore, when we comb our hair, the popping sound that one customarily hears is the literal breaking off of the hair follicle making it weaker. As the authors correctly note, *"Strictly speaking our hair should not be combed."* [6] This is especially true if we attempt to use combs designed for combing the hair of Europeans, Asians and others who have straight hair. Their type of hair lacks the weaving affect found in the African's hair, and when combed, yields no popping sound or breakage of hair. This points to the fact that African people have erroneously adopted the use of European combs and brushes for grooming their hair. In other words, to use European combs and brushes to groom African hair is not the wise or correct choice of tools for grooming our type of hair. They were not designed for use with our hair.

The hair of most Africans is coiled or spiraled in texture. When we speak of African hair, we specifically refer to what some pejoratively call "kinky," "nappy," or "knotty" hair. More correctly, this type of hair has a very tight curl, and the weaving affect already spoken of is readily apparent to most from mere observation. The textures may range from very tight curls to nearly straight. Much of the straight hair found in those Blacks who have "naturally straight" curls is most commonly a result of the enslavement our ancestors endured.[7] Due to the enslavement, millions of African women were brutally raped by the Europeans and Arabs who enslaved our ancestors. Thus, there are many Africans, as a result of these unholy encounters, whose hair texture is of a mixed quality. This texture of hair may be passed from one generation to the next in varying degrees. We are concerned here with those who have the tighter curl but attempt to "rid" themselves of it by some artificial means *(chemicals, hot-combs, etc.)*.

African hair is very beautiful to the eye and to the touch. It is the natural adornment of the other physical features of Africans. It accents our shapely noses and lips. It matches and compliments our complexions. Its touch is not offensive but warm and comfortable, bidding us to linger in its embrace a moment longer. It crowns our entire body in royalty, and it affirms our humanity. We love to play in it and be creative with it because not only is it flexible, but it is also diverse. We may decide to wear it in a short natural, cutting it into some unique design or shape. We may braid it into any of the thousands of styles we already know, or we may create new ones. We may choose to cut it all off for that clean cool look while retaining our masculinity or our femininity. Some choose to simply wash and oil it letting it grow into beautiful locks. Others may even choose to straighten it, but this method usually kills it. Such unlimited variety could not be exhausted in a lifetime. No other people on the planet can boast of having so many hair options available to them. Yet, the majority of Black women choose only to straighten their hair! Why they do this is no secret when we begin to understand the psychological impact enslavement, colonialism and racism has had on African peoples.

Ghosts from the Old Plantation: The Impact of Enslavement

Many who are unaware of the damage enslavement inflicted on the African psyche may be heard arguing they have the freedom of choice to wear their hair straight or however they may choose. This is true. We acknowledge there is freedom of choice, but we question why the majority of Black women exclusively and solely choose to straighten their hair when so many other alternatives are available to them. It would seem that if they were really exercising freedom of choice, we would see more diverse natural hairstyles among Black women. As it stands, however, roughly 80% or more of the African women in America, for example, wear their hair straight from the time they are old enough until the time they die. Rarely, if ever, do they remotely consider wearing any form of their natural hair, and it is not even considered as an option. If it were truly a matter of freedom of choice, we should expect to see different percentages with regard to those wearing naturals versus those choosing to straighten their hair; e.g., 35% with braids, 40% with naturals, 15% with locks, and 10% with straightened hair.

The haunting reality, nevertheless, leaves us with a sad commentary. The negative terms often used when discussing African hair or Black hair betrays the freedom of choice argument as superficial and lacking real substance. No other people on the face of the earth is more collectively obsessed with altering their natural hair as are Black women, and no other group collectively thinks of and speaks of their hair in the derogative terms we are all familiar with in our community among both men and women.

This is not a put down of these women, for we recognize that there are no other women in the world who have endured and suffered as much as African women, but it represents an analysis of the sickness/illness resulting from the damage enslavement, colonialism and racism inflicted upon us as a people inasmuch as we all have condoned and accepted this abnormal behavior to one degree or another.

We have been made to think of our unique hair as something to be ashamed of, and we go to dangerous lengths to alter it. Although attempts to alter our hair is more evident among Black women than among Black men, there are a small percentage of Black men who attempt to alter their natural hair. This is especially true of many men in the entertainment field. The majority of Black men, however, wear their hair in some natural form, and Black women usually expect and even demand that they do. This is as it should be. Those few who do alter their natural hair are usually seen as peculiar and may even incur ridicule from African women. Again, this is as it should be. In fact, men who artificially alter their hair turn off many Black women. Our sisters should not expect to be held to a lesser standard.

The extreme measures which Black men have used to alter their hair more recently but for shorter durations have been the perm or relaxer and the "scary" curl better known as the jerri curl in its many manifestations. Earlier forms include the process or conk and the pressed wave. The pressed wave look is perhaps the most reoccurring attempt by African men to alter their hair and the most widely acceptable abnormal procedure. This is due to the fact that we have been conditioned to value "wavy" or "curly" textured hair because it is regarded as "good hair," which when translated means the "best" hair. This type of hair is usually perceived as a prized asset in the opposite sex. We, however, maintain that it is an aberration and a deviation from the African aesthetic especially since it devalues those who do not have this texture of hair. The value emphasis of "good hair" is not on the quality of the person but places a high premium on a distorted perception of an asset. This does not mean that those who do not have this texture of hair are any less valuable.

To attribute a person's worth to their grade or texture of hair is ridiculous and subjects one to building upon a faulty foundation. It is superficial and it is anti-African. For too long we have been imposed upon with this type of foolishness by White people's standards wherein value judgments were made about a person's character or abilities based on hair texture or skin tone. We are merely pointing out that African hair, your hair, whatever the texture, is beautiful and glorious just as it is!!

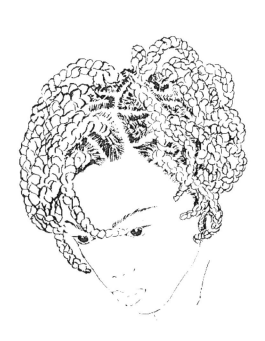

A mind attacked and conquered is guided easily away from the paths of its own soul.

— Ayi Kwei Armah —

And on top of my head was this thick, smooth sheen of shining red hair as straight as any white man's . . . This was the first really big step toward self degradation: when I endured all of that pain, literally burning my flesh to have it look like a white man's hair. I had joined that multitude of Negro men and women in America who are brainwashed into believing that the black people are 'inferior' and white people 'superior' that they will even violate and mutilate their God-created bodies to try to look 'pretty' by white standards.

— Malcolm X —

Chapter 2

The Destruction of Black Hair

In order to properly understand the present, we must study the past. This allows us to intelligently shape the future. If we want to better understand why Black people love to hate their hair, we must look to the past for more correct answers. Having done so, we will have information that shapes our future thinking and ultimately influence our behavior.

The kidnapping and enslavement that our ancestors encountered was designed and modeled, perhaps unwittingly, after a parent-child relationship. Our people were treated like children, and Whites (kidnappers) regarded themselves as parents. In this capacity, Whites provided food, clothing and shelter, albeit at the basic or survival level. In this diabolical relationship, our ancestors, in the role of children, behaved in ways just as children do with their parents. The kidnappers would determine who would marry whom and when. They would settle disputes between our enslaved ancestors just as parents resolve disputes between quarreling siblings. Our ancestors were not the ones primarily concerned with providing the needs of their own children because the white enslavers provided the necessities of life for them and their children. In addition, the kidnappers, if they saw fit and as they saw fit in their own best interest, could, would, and did sell off the child/children of our ancestors to other Whites, which resulted in the destruction of many African families.

When our ancestors became sick, it was the responsibility of the white kidnappers to provide medical attention. When our ancestors became "unruly" or committed some act unacceptable to the enslaver, they, like a parent, would "chastise" them. So in these ways we see a parent-child type of relationship (a grossly distorted one), which lasted for centuries from one generation to the next.

The impact on the minds of African people was devastating and, with the passage of time, the damage became almost imperceptible.

In such a setup, it is not surprising that many of our ancestors, like children, attempted to imitate their white enslaver. This emulation was evident in deed, in word, and in appearance since it is a natural response for children to aspire to be like their parents. Those who possessed lighter complexions and hair more like the Whites (those who were the offspring of White men who raped Black women) were usually treated a little better and many of them regarded themselves as being better than the other Blacks. Concerning this point, clinical psychologist Na'im Akbar indicates the following:

> *Only those persons who looked-like, acted-liked, and thought in the framework of reference of the master*[kidnapper], *were completely acceptable. Those earning such acceptance were projected as far superior to those who looked-like, acted-like, and thought in the frame of reference of African self-affirmation.* [1]

Those in this last group were especially prone to imitating Whites. Thus, rewards and punishments were apportioned based upon one's capitulation to White people's standards. This sent a clear message to the other Africans that they would receive better treatment from Whites if they too, could approximate the Whites in appearance. They would also be treated better and held in higher esteem by other Africans if they were light skinned with "wavy hair."

The Results of A Distorted Relationship

In response, many of our people began to find ways to accomplish this. They tried to lighten their skin; still prevalent in our communities today in clever but transparent disguise. They tried to make their lips thin like Whites and to make their noses like the Whites or longed for these attributes. Now that plastic surgeons are able to perform these procedures, many of our people are spending the last of their hard earned dollars to receive their "white disguise" by this method. This merely points to the deeply imbedded self-hatred too many of us have of our physical features. It is plainly the outward manifestations of the inner contempt that reveals what we really think of ourselves.

One of the most glaring and publicized contemporary cases in point was the late entertainer, Michael Jackson. Whether or not Michael Jackson had the skin disorder he professed, it was apparent that he had some latent contempt for Black features. The surgical work he had done to his lips and nose had nothing to do with his skin disorder. Neither did it have any connection with his jerri curl or relaxed hairstyle. Yet, he only did what many Africans would do if they had the money and the chance. In fact, for decades many Blacks have been secretly engaging in the very activity they accuse and ridiculed him of doing. One need only to check the advertisements in some of the old magazines *(early to mid 20th century)* marketed toward African Americans and by African Americans. There you will see an abundance of advertisements for hair straighteners and skin lighteners. They still exist in American magazines of the 21st century, but in more subtle and sophisticated forms. On the other hand, in various parts of Africa, an abundance of more blatant forms of such advertisements still grace the pages of many magazines.

The apex of this absurd behavior, however, finds its most completed and most accepted practice in straightening the hair so that it looks as much as possible like White people's hair or at the least Africans with wavy or straight hair textures. *The parent-child relationship created during our enslavement remains with us today but in a more insidious and diabolical form.* Much of this activity has to do with Black people attempting to receive approval and acceptance from Whites and an attempt to boost their self-esteem and status in our own communities.

The Beginning of the End for Black Hair

Before being kidnapped and taken from the continent of Africa to be enslaved, Black women and men did many marvelous and creative things with their hair. They braided and plaited it in a variety of shapes and styles, which varied from group to group. Some wore their hair in short naturals while others wore longer naturals. Others wore their hair in locks. Still others shaved their head donning the bald look. Sonja Peterson-Lewis cites Willie Lee Morrow on this point as follows:

> *In Africa, the curly/kinky hair was looked upon grandly, faithfully cared for and painstakingly decorated. Exotic hairstyles were not only common, but were the norm, for there were centuries of tradition behind hair decoration, hair design... The African's hairstyle often reflected his and her tribal customs. Many of the ancient tribesmen created hairstyles which today's stylists cannot comprehend.* [2]

When we observe African people on the continent of Africa and in the Diaspora today, we see some of these various styles. Before the enslavement, we had not been afflicted with the self-hatred evidenced by later generations of Blacks (whether on the continent, in the Americas or in the Caribbean islands) who have been bombarded by a system of white supremacy that glorifies the physical features of Whites including their hair, while denigrating and ridiculing the hair and other physical features of Blacks. This, combined with the psychological indoctrination of the white-is-right concept and the white-god image, left a deep and harmful impression on the psyche of Black people.

African women and men used different types of techniques and tools to style their hair before being kidnapped and subjected to the horrific enslavement experience in what to the whites was dubbed the "New World." The techniques were not lost in this transition but the tools were. This is of crucial importance because although they remembered how to care for their hair when they arrived at the various locations in the Americas, they did not have the familiar and necessary tools to groom their hair. This in turn created problems of untold proportions since these were a people who placed much value upon personal and group appearance. The cultures from which they were kidnapped placed significant value on personal cleanliness and grooming. Yet, this new and hellish situation did not attribute the same value to Blacks regarding their personal well-being or appearance except as it related to the profit motive. Na'im Akbar points out the following:

The slaves were kept filthy and the very nature of physical restraints over long periods of time began to develop in the people a sense of their helplessness. The loss of the ability to even clean one's body and to shield oneself (SIC) from a blow began to teach the slave that he should have no self-respect. [3]

Regarding this issue, Peterson-Lewis asserts:

The same filthy conditions that affected and afflicted their bodies also affected their hair. The Africans, part of a tradition steeped in the art and science of highly specialized hair care, arrived this (SIC) time in the Western world with a scalp that was often infested with sores, and hair that was matted and soiled with perspiration, blood, feces, urine and dirt, and all this without a proper comb. [4]

The Right Tools For Our Hair - Lost

Consequently, they were never provided with the necessary tools and materials needed to groom their unique hair. Needless to say, when our people were kidnapped from the continent, they were not afforded the privilege of packing their personal belongings, which would have included hair-grooming tools. Peterson-Lewis describes the African comb in the following terms:

Combs having wide, rounded teeth befitting the curly structure of African hair were carved from hard wood or ivory. The teeth were strong and perfectly rounded and spaced so that they would neither snag the African's tightly coiled hair nor pierce the scalp. The predecessor of the 'picks' that appeared in the West during the revolution of the natural in the 1960s, these traditional combs were not only functional; they were also often works of art, having been decoratively and expertly carved for the individuals who would use them. [5]

Even if they somehow managed to bring one of these combs, it would have inevitably been lost before our ancestors were forced onto the waiting ships. It must be remembered that their lives and the lives of their loved ones were at stake. Thus, the preservation of life was top priority and left little or no room for concern over hair tools.

Upon arrival in the "New World," everything about the African and Africa came under an insidiously diabolical attack and condemnation. All of our physical features, our complexion, our nose, our lips, our buttocks, and our hair suffered continuous and severe contempt, mockery and derision. Contrary to the facts, Africa was intentionally projected as an uncivilized, undeveloped and barbaric place. These lies were told not to the first generation of enslaved Africans but to the generations of Africans that were born into the evils of enslavement. Obviously, these lies would not have affected those who were newly arrived from the continent since they knew the truth, knew the reality of their homeland and valued their own aesthetics. It would have been useless for the enslavers to attempt this with the first generation of Africans. With subsequent generations, however, it was an altogether different story.

The Subject Nobody Wants to Talk About

Those who enslaved us imposed their diabolical schemes on our ancestors of the ensuing generations while they were children. In other words, they directed and focused their evil intentions on our ancestors when they were innocent and defenseless children. These children, the focus of the attack, were told that they were ugly; their noses were too big; their lips were too large; their skin was a curse from God; their buttocks were too broad; that they descended from savages in the so-called "wilds" of Africa and that their hair was ugly and abnormal.

In other words, the message that the white kidnapping enslavers wanted to convey to these children was that they were not valuable; that they did not matter; that they were abnormal and unacceptable as they naturally came into the world. The children, having no defense against these satanic lies, internalized the messages and grew up with a budding self-contempt and self-hatred that was passed from one generation to the next. Those children believed the lies, and when they grew up, they passed those same messages and those same lies, with a mega dose of contempt, to their own children.

Whites, in an attempt to create the illusion or the idea that they were supreme beings and the standard by which all others should be measured, set in motion a diabolical anti-African, anti-Black sentiment in both Blacks and Whites. This became a self-perpetuating idea and practice, which manifested itself into a tenacious African self-hatred in which some of our ancestors unwittingly, participated.

Today, we are the descendants of those children, one of those latter generations, and we, too many of us, unwittingly and ignorantly pass the same message, the same lies in full bloom to our children in a multiplicity of ways. These lies and messages are so deeply imbedded in our psyche that most of us have never even given it a first thought let alone a second thought as to their origin or their impact on us. This is, in part, why some of us may be heard justifying why we straighten our hair with such phrases as: *"It's my freedom of choice," "It's the style,"* and *"It's easier to manage,"* etc. Or by saying, *"I might straighten my hair, but I know who I am."*

Yet, we don't discuss it. Women don't discuss it. Men don't discuss it. We all sit silently by while our mothers, sisters, aunts, wives, girlfriends, and daughters converge in "beauty shops" and neighborhood kitchens to engage in one of the most self-contemptuous and untoward activities imaginable—imitating White people by straightening their hair. The "we" refers to all of us —men, women, elderly, youth, the educated and the not so educated and the religious of every persuasion in our community. We all give tacit approval to this activity, and by our silence we condone the behavior and thus, make the unacceptable acceptable.

Looking Back To See Straight

It is important to remember that when enslavement of Black people ended, there was not a period of readjustment or healing to help us correct the lies and notions of self-hatred that had been created and instilled into us. We, in fact, walked out of physical slavery in a state of mental slavery. We were physically "free" but mentally shackled with the lies about ourselves that were created about us during enslavement. That mentality has lasted from 1865 to the present.

Also worthy of mention, ironically, is the fact that the first Black woman to become a millionaire in this country did so by creating and marketing products to help Black women straighten their hair. That woman was Madam C. J. Walker, a business and marketing genius. Although her intentions were noble *(to help Black women feel good and beautiful in a society that did not value them or their beauty)*, she misguidedly helped reinforce the notion of their inferiority.

The complicity and participation of Black men in this cover-up needs to be highlighted. Many Black men condone and even demand that our women have their hair straightened to feed their clandestine desire for the look of White women in Black women. They have also been conditioned by the enslavement experience and its aftermath regarding this activity.

Many Black men even ridicule sisters for wearing their hair natural or for desiring to wear it natural. Of course, this contributes to the continuation of hair straightening on the part of sisters in order to please their "men" whether it is their father, husband, or boyfriend. These unjust demands by African men help contribute to the destruction of our hair.

The Root of the Problem

When our people were subjected to the condemnation and attack on their physical features as evidenced during enslavement, their hair, a peculiarity to Whites, was deemed inferior and became an object of ridicule and scorn. For African women who came from a tradition where women were adored and held in high esteem, this was a devastating blow. Subject to feelings of personal inadequacy, constant humiliation, and repeated rape, her hair became a burden as well as a symbol of what characterized her alleged inferiority. Without proper tools to groom their unique hair, Black women, during enslavement, kept their hair covered with a bandanna to avoid embarrassment. In fact, the bandanna became a common adornment for them during this period. [6]

It is common knowledge that Black women during the enslavement were the primary caretakers of White children, which included grooming their hair. This close contact impacted their perceptions of Whites and themselves. The society was already shot through with the white-is-right concept; that to be white or near white was to be valuable and worthwhile, but to be Black or African was to be antithetical, anathematized, devalued and worthless. These women and men thus came to view being White, and the privileges accompanying it, as positive and being Black as negative — something to be avoided at all costs.

Why is the Comb a Problem?

Believe it or not, the instrument used to groom White people's hair is, in part, the culprit. The comb, which was designed specifically for and is most suitable for grooming White people's hair or straight hair, proves demonic when used on African hair due to the unique structure of our hair.

Black women, without tools made specifically for grooming their hair, began using combs made for straight hair. This resulted in horror and pain. It would not work.

Instead of smoothly gliding through the multiple strands of hair without a "snag" as it did when combing the hair of Whites, the comb became a torturous weapon that caught itself in a web of tangled African hair that would not surrender to the insistent demands of a foreign intrusion in its midst.

47

When and if the subject of hair straightening is broached, we hear attempts to justify it with faulty reasoning due to lack of understanding the enslavement experience and not having an understanding of its continued impact upon our behavior today. Enslavement, with its beastly brutality and untold horrors, also carried with it the most diabolical form of brainwashing any people have ever experienced in the history of humanity. Self-hatred has no equal in the realm of human activity. But this is exactly what those who enslaved our ancestors were bent on accomplishing, the hatred of the African image by the Africans themselves and by the rest of the world. We know that it was successful as seen in the way we as African people contemptuously regard our physical features, especially our hair. Haki Madhubuti's words sum this up cogently:

> *For a Black person to actively, all of his or her life, seek to be white is the ultimate in irrational and psychotic behavior. Yet, to be and seek values of whiteness has been the foundation of most of our education, so in essense (SIC) we only do what we have been taught to do. The normal seeking the abnormal.* [7]

The brainwashing to which we have been subjected has bounded and shackled us more tenaciously and insidiously than physical shackles could ever hope to achieve. Our mind, like a bird, has been caught in the midst of flight and must be liberated. Only then will we come to the realization that the behavior we term as normal concerning our hair is in actuality abnormal behavior. It demonstrates an intense internal yearning to be White, or as near White as one can get, by any means possible. It is also indicative of a continued sense of being inferior to Whites. As Akbar correctly asserts,

...our persistent and futile efforts to look like and act like Caucasian people, is based upon this sense of inferiority. The persistent tendency to think of dark skin as unattractive, kinky hair as 'bad' hair, and African features as less appealing than Caucasian features, come from this sense of inferiority. [8]

The destruction of Black hair has more to do with the way we think about it... rather than... what we do to it. Whatever we do to it and how we speak of it... is a result of... our thinking about it.

When we change our thinking about our hair, we will also change our actions toward it. Action is the outgrowth, the result, or the evidence of our thinking. Since we *think* that Black hair is ugly, difficult to manage, unattractive, and unacceptable, we act accordingly. Our action confirms our thinking that our hair is actually ugly. When we change our thinking about our hair, when we begin to see it as beautiful, pretty, and attractive, we will also begin to appreciate it and wear it naturally. Only then will others see its beauty and begin to accept it.

For seasons and seasons and seasons all our movement has been a going against our self, a journey into our killers' desire.

— Ayi Kwei Armah —

It is the basis of the image which is the ground of a man's [or woman's] acts. This is a point of enormous importance, for men [and women] act out of their image. They respond not to the situation but to the situation transformed by the images they carry in their minds. In short, they respond to the image-situation, to the ideas they have of themselves in the situation . . . and if you want to change a situation, you have to change the image men [and women] have of themselves and of their situation.

— Lerone Bennett, Jr. —

Chapter 3

The Straight Hair Fantasy

Due to the psychological brainwashing already discussed, it should be understood that many Black women will go to great lengths to straighten their hair and to keep it straightened for as long as possible so that it does not "go back." Little Black girls are "groomed" from the time they are old enough to walk to look forward to the day when they will get their first relaxer. The message sent to these children at a very early age is that their natural hair is not acceptable; it is not normal for them to be who they really are.

Adults send conflicting messages when they tell children to be proud of who they are when they themselves are guilty of having altered their natural hair. Many women would be lost for an answer to the question, *"Mommy, why do you straighten your hair?"* It is said that action speaks louder than words, and it is commonly accepted that children listen not to what we say, but what we do. These women are in fact, only perpetuating what their mothers did to them as children.

How The Media Affects Images of Black Hair

Black magazines and television commercials now boldly advertise hair relaxers targeted specifically toward little African girls. If their hair is not straightened chemically, then the alternative is hot combing the child's hair. Either way, the end result is to produce a head of hair they think is free of "naps" making it easier to comb using the European's comb. In reality, however, these procedures also destroy the natural beauty of African hair.

The images that we are constantly bombarded with on television, in magazines, and on billboards and social media platforms, aid in giving us a negative view not only of the natural state of our hair but our other features as well. Standards of beauty depicted in these media portray tall and thin Caucasian models with long, flowing hair, usually blonde. The occasional Black woman in these media will also usually have "long flowing hair" (maybe even blonde).

African-Americans spend many hours watching television and scrolling through social media platforms. When one is subjected to a daily, hour-by-hour diet of these visual images, it is easy to understand why many men and women of African ancestry continue to view their God-given features as ugly or bad. Where are the images of black men and women with African features? Because this is an unusual occurrence on television and other media, many Blacks view their African features as strange, weird, and worst yet, as ugly. We must empower ourselves by producing images of ourselves, not after those which fit into a Eurocentric standard of beauty but those which properly represent Black people and the beautiful features we possess.

Young Black directors such as Ryan Coogler of *Black Panther* fame and actor/producer Jordan Peele's productions of movies such as *Get Out*, *Us*, and the new *Twilight Zone* series are casting more black women with natural hair styles. For example, in the Black Panther movie, which consisted of a large cast of women, all the women wore natural hair styles of one sort or another. Peele, in his productions, tends to cast Black women who wear their hair in natural styles, too. Their efforts and that of many other young directors and producers in this area are worthy of support.

Although there are only a handful of African magazines on the market, the majority of Black models used in these magazines possess European features —light eyes, light skin, and of course, long, straightened hair. In recent years, more Black magazines have begun to feature a more diverse group of models with a variety of natural hair styles. Many white established magazines are also following suit. These are developments headed in the right direction because young Black girls get to see more positive examples of themselves in the media. Yet, it is only the tip of the iceberg.

Since the first edition of this book in 1996, there has been, as we predicted, a rise in Black women wearing natural hairstyles. That has given rise to seeing more Black women wearing natural hairstyles in television commercials and programs, billboards and movies, and social media. We applaud these developments but recognize that there is still more work to be done because large numbers of Black women, especially younger Black women 25 and under, continue to straighten their hair and use excessive straight weaves. Additionally, another adverse phenomena that has developed is the rise of many Black women and girls wearing wigs. Some of them wear wigs because (1) their hair, due to continued use of harsh chemicals, has been damaged beyond recovery or (2) they are dealing with a variety of health issues. Both of these groups wear wigs out of necessity. Even more disturbing are the large number of women wearing straight wigs who have a full head of healthy hair! More alarming is that many in this category have gone natural but still succumb to this practice. It is another factor that points to the psychological issues surrounding our hair. Many are still not fully comfortable with their own natural hair even though they are aware of the benefits and freedom it provides.

Hair Fantasy Land

Despite the advances that have been made in the last twenty years, in this Eurocentric society, the "natural African" hairstyle is still looked upon by many Blacks and Whites as being "unnatural," whereas artificially straightened hair is looked upon as being "natural." There is something grossly wrong with that assessment! It is a fantasy. *Whites live in the fantasy that their type of hair, straight hair, is the best hair; the standard for everyone else. Blacks live in the fantasy that this is indeed true.* We maintain that all people of African ancestry must reassess the prejudices against themselves of which they may or may not be aware, and channel that energy to the uplifting and glorification of their natural, God-given physical features.

Ironically, many of the features we reject in ourselves are the very features that people of other ethnic groups admire about us and try to emulate. For example, we now see White women undergoing surgery in order to have large voluptuous lips like African women and lying in the sun or visiting tanning salons to get darker complexions. We understand these acts, and we are flattered that they want to be or look like us (though they may not admit this). When we imitate them by straightening our hair, they too are flattered that we want to look like them (though we may not want to admit it).

The Other Little Nasty "N" Word

Hair is a very popular topic among Black women. If you engage in conversation with them or overhear them discussing their hair, you will notice that the word "nappy" and other negative terms will be used several times within a sentence to describe the state of their hair. This applies to all age groups from little girls to grown women. The word is even more frequently used when the woman is due for a "touch-up." This means that it is time to get another relaxer. The "new growth," as it is referred to, which starts from the scalp, as it emerges looks distinctly different from the ends of the hair, which is still straightened. For the sisters who straighten their hair this is almost like the end of the world. In their mind, if it is not straight, then it is ugly and not appealing to the eye.

To add insult to injury, the uninformed spouse or boyfriend will sometimes ask the sister when is she going to get her hair "done" (as in cooked) because it is "nappy."

Once, a conversation between two adolescent African-American girls discussing the condition of their hair was overheard. They must have used the word "nappy" five or more times between the two of them. This discussion is not the exception but the rule, and it typifies the way we have been conditioned to view our natural hair.

We refer to nappy as the "N" word because we should not apply this word in a negative sense to describe our hair. What exactly does this word mean? The Webster's New Collegiate Dictionary, 1977, defines "nappy," when used as an adjective, as "kinky." Kinky is defined by the same dictionary as "closely twisted or curled (as it relates to hair); bizarre and outlandish; far out." Interestingly, *The New Webster's Comprehensive Dictionary of the English Language,* 1991, defines nappy as a "baby's diaper." There is no reference made connecting nappy with the state of one's hair in the updated dictionary. The Merriam-Webster online dictionary agrees with both these definitions.[1] The term has not changed over the years.

This dictionary defines kinky, however, as "having kinks" (*esp. of hair*). Often, people of African ancestry will refer to the hair, which is located closest to the nape of the neck (the kitchen) and the hair around the hairline as "naps," but it may also refer to the hair on the entire head. What are naps? The latter dictionary defines naps as, "the soft, fuzzy surface on cloth or wool material." The word is not negative in and of itself, but the images associated with the word — bad and ugly hair— are negative. Why then is naps used so negatively?

The natural texture of African hair is spiraled or coiled. There is nothing negative, bad, or ugly about this type of hair except as White people have defined it in relation to their hair and as Blacks have accepted their incorrect conclusion. That Blacks in fact accept it in negative terms is evident by the overwhelming number of Black women who straighten their hair and by the negative way in which they speak of their own natural hair.

Men and women of African descent use many other adjectives to put down and degrade the natural state of their beautiful hair. Words such as knotty, woolly, peasy, and kinky are used extensively. The continued use of these words reflect the negative image they have regarding their hair.

It is also interesting that women who wear natural hairstyles are not exempt from using nappy and other negative words to describe their hair. Just because a person wears natural hair does not necessarily mean they think their hair is beautiful. This also includes Black men who speak negatively about our natural hair. Remnants of the psychological damage done to us during and after enslavement and colonialism still exists, and it may take many years for us to extricate ourselves from the use of these derogative terms. We must make a conscious and concerted effort to eliminate the word "nappy" and all other words associated with it from our vocabulary so that future generations will not even know that such words existed as it pertains to our hair. If, however, one feels absolutely compelled to use the term "nappy," we suggest that it be used in a positive sense instead of one that is negative.

Revealing The Goldie Locks Syndrome: "Good Hair"/ "Bad Hair?"

The discussion of African hair would be incomplete if no mention was made of the "good hair vs. bad hair" issue or the Goldie locks syndrome that is so prevalent in Black communities. If your ancestral background is heavily mixed with European ancestry, it is possible that your hair will closely resemble the hair of the European. It will be naturally straight, or it may be curly, though not fully resembling the curl of the more tightly coiled African hair, but that of the European. This also applies to those who may have Indian or Hispanic heritage. African men and women erroneously refer to this kind of hair as "good hair." Those with this type of hair, men and women, are usually valued more in our communities. This is because it approximates the hair of Whites, and since western society values the European aesthetic and not the African aesthetic, we perpetuate their standards.

On the other hand, if your hair is tightly curled, short, and coarse, Blacks tend to refer to this type of hair as "bad hair." This is due in part to the subconscious contempt many Black people have toward their hair, and it also highlights our general ignorance regarding the care and maintenance of our natural hair.

How do Black men perceive all of this? Regretfully, many Black men will not even look at a Black woman with short, and/or what they perceive as "bad hair." They prefer and actually seek women who have lighter skin. It is a real "bonus" if that woman also has long, straight hair. If the woman does, however, have dark skin, then it is almost imperative that she have straight hair, preferably long, to go along with "that" complexion. What does this do to the psyche of the Black woman whose hair is short, "coarse," and/or "nappy" as she perceives it? She will be on a continual mission throughout her life to keep her hair artificially straightened so that her man will be pacified.

This also applies to light-skinned women who have the tightly curled African hair, but her skin usually compensates for this "shortcoming" as some of the brothers may see it.

Fortunately, more Black men are starting to reevaluate this phenomenon, and are beginning to appreciate the regality that is exhibited by women who wear their hair in natural styles and even encourage them to do so. We hope these numbers continue to increase.

How do Black women perceive the hair of Black men? This issue could get very complicated. There are, of course, some Black women who seek Black men with so-called "good hair." Again, there is a real "bonus" if that man has light skin and/or European features.

But how do Black women perceive Black men with chemically straightened hair? From our life experiences and through conversations with Black women, we found that most of these women preferred a Black man with NO CHEMICALS in his hair. They prefer that Black men wear their hair in its natural state. To put a chemical straightener or "curl" in their hair would make Black men appear too artificial, thus, unattractive to most Black women. Of course, there is a double standard here! Why does this not apply to Black women as well? Why is she not perceived as appearing artificial when she straightens her hair?

In reality, there is no such thing as good hair or bad hair except as we attempt to define it in relationship to White people's hair. It is a foolish notion. They are not our standard of measurement. In the traditional African value system good was not determined by one's assets or physical features, but by the character of the person and their actions. Dr. Molefi K. Asante in discussing Afrocentric values asserts, *"If a person's actions are not good, it does not matter how the person looks physically. Doing good is equivalent to being beautiful."* [2]

The notion of us having good or bad hair is a fantasy, and to describe it or speak of it in such terms causes us to devalue our own people. It is divisive and detrimental to both the individual and the community. Some men and women in our communities have often chosen their life's mate based on the premise of their features, including their hair, resembling those of Europeans/Whites. They (Whites) started this absurdity to convince us that they were superior, but it is incumbent upon us to refute the lie and reconstruct and restore our full humanity. We are all valuable and beautiful in our community regardless of the hair texture we possess.

Chemical Hair Relaxing and Thermal Hair Straightening (Hair Pressing)

According to one of the definitive cosmetology textbooks, Milady's Standard Textbook of Cosmetology (1991), the definition of chemical hair relaxing is as follows: *"The process of permanently rearranging the basic structure of overly curly hair into a straight form. When done professionally, it leaves the hair straight and in a satisfactory condition to be set in almost any style."* *(Emphasis ours)* When one reads this definition, there are all kinds of negative subtleties involved. For instance, the reference to curly hair as being "overly curly" gives one the impression that there is something wrong or unnatural about hair that is tightly curled, i.e. African hair.

This reveals that others outside our communities have decided, in comparison to their hair, that our hair is "overly curly." That is unacceptable and untrue. (A proper assessment, from our view, could conclude that their hair is under curly and not fully developed compared to ours.) This also suggests that something is abnormal about Black folk's hair. The phrase, *"Leaving the hair in a satisfactory condition"* also has negative implications. In a "satisfactory condition" means by European standards not by African standards. This definition alone leads one to believe that straight hair is superior and that African hair is inferior. It is no wonder African women are so confused about their hair! By these and other subtle ways, those who style Black women's hair are imbued with further contempt for natural hair beyond the other negative ideas they have picked up from the society and the historical development. The training they receive as exemplified by Milady's and other cosmetology textbooks makes it necessary. They buy into this cultural imposition almost without question. Therefore, it is no small wonder that those stylists so trained would not be the ones, in most cases, to broach the subject of why Black women straighten their hair.

The difference between thermal hair straightening (hot combing), flat ironing, whose use is more recent, and chemical relaxing is that when the hair is washed, it reverts back to its original, natural state (much to the chagrin of many Black women). This procedure is even more negatively defined by Milady's Standard Textbook of Cosmetology where it states: *"When properly done, hair pressing temporarily straightens overly curly or unruly hair."*(Emphasis ours) What constitutes "unruly hair?" Is unruly hair considered to be "nappy hair?" According to this statement, African hair is characterized as "unruly." This conclusion is based on the standards of White folk's hair, which we have all too willingly accepted as the standard of measurement. The definition further states, *"a good hair pressing leaves the hair in a natural and lustrous condition…"* This is absurd, contradictory, untrue, and unacceptable! How could pressing out the "natural" curl in your hair leave it in a "natural" condition? This is the type of education and thinking that tends to prevail, and it is a fantasy to which we as a people have thoroughly succumbed.

The minds of African people are still crowded with the image of Europeans as superior beings.
—Marimba Ani—

Self-hatred and low self-esteem
Non-existent love within a hollow and shell-shocked soul
Color contact lenses, Bleach cremes and nose jobs
Lipo-suction spirit killing techniques designed to maim and destroy. War crimes committed against the souls of a people.
—Sisters Griots—

Chapter 4

Mirror, Mirror On The Wall…

We surveyed groups of Black women who straighten their hair in various occupations ranging from ages 14-50 (see form in appendix). Educational backgrounds ranged from not having a high school diploma to the post-graduate level. A list of general reasons Black women give for straightening their hair was provided. The respondents were asked to check one or more reasons that applied only to themselves. A section was added for the respondents to add any reason that was not listed. In the next section of the questionnaire, the respondents were asked to rate in order of importance the most important reason to the least important reason for straightening their hair. (This was to be done only if they checked more than one reason). The results were interesting.

Opinion Poll: Black Women *Straighten* Their Hair Because...

Over half of the participants, 67%, responded that the reason they *straighten* their hair is because it is easier to manage. 80% of these women rated this reason as the most important reason why they straighten their hair.

Interestingly, 47% of the participants responded that they had never given any thought as to why they straighten their hair. Over half of those participants however, 57%, rated this as the number one reason why they straighten their hair.

Surprisingly, only 20% of the women polled responded that "it was the style, and everyone else straightens their hair." 33% of those participants listed this as the most important reason. None of the participants indicated that their boyfriend/spouse preferred their hair straight. Only 1% of participants responded that straight hair looked better, that their employer would look unfavorably at a natural style, and that natural hair was unattractive.

Nearly 27% of the participants listed other reasons for straightening their hair. A few of them were:

✦ *"You can do a lot more with relaxed hair."*
✦ *"My mother has been straightening my hair since I was little."*
✦ *"If I had a natural style, I would only wear it short, and I would be locked into one style."*

From these results, it is evident that the majority of the women polled felt that it is easier to manage straight hair.

This is due in part to the lack of knowledge and information regarding the care and maintenance of their own natural hair. [1] We maintain that if these women were to wear their hair in a natural style for just a short period of time, it would become quite evident which style, straight or natural, would be easier to manage.

Perhaps the most disturbing result of this poll is the fact that a large majority of the women had *never given any thought as to why* they put chemicals in their hair or why they straighten it. Evidence has clearly shown that when not used properly, and in some cases when used properly, chemical straighteners can have devastating effects on both the scalp and health of some people. Many Black women will spend their entire lives putting something unnatural into their hair and never give a moment's thought as to why they do it and what the consequences of their actions may produce.

"But I Won't Get a Job If I Wear My Hair Natural…"

Over time we have spoken to and read about many Black women who wear natural hairstyles in the workplace. A few revealed to us that they were covertly and overtly asked to straighten their hair when they reported to work so that they would fit into what the employer considered "white beauty standards." Some have even been ridiculed and fired because they wore natural hair styles. A quick Internet search will bring up recently reported news articles and commentaries detailing these employment issues concerning Blacks and natural hairstyles in the workplace.

In conducting hair seminars, lectures, and in the course of general conversations, we have found that the issue of employment and natural hair will inevitably come up. It is usually concluded that wearing natural hair in the workplace would not be looked upon favorably. This rationale is not without some justification given the historical realities of white cultural hegemony and economic strength. We contend, however, that if this is the only reason used for straightening one's hair, it is not as strong a reason as it may appear on the surface.

It smacks of expecting to receive permission from White folks to wear your natural hair. This is reminiscent of the parent/child relationship created between Blacks and Whites during our enslavement. Thus, it is easier to understand why many women are reluctant to wear their hair natural—their "white parents" disapprove. In other words, if you really want to wear your hair natural, nothing and no one can stop you, except you. If you are the only Black person in your workplace wearing natural hair, there is virtue in being the "first one!" IT HAS TO START SOMEWHERE AND WITH SOMEONE! **Moreover, to ask or insist that Black women wear their hair straight or altered in order to be accepted in ANY workplace (or other parts of the society for that matter) represents the height of racism/white supremacy!!** What is equally appalling is our capitulation to and acceptance of this absurd demand.

It is not accepted or expected that one *must* change the color of one's eyes or the color of one's skin in order to obtain employment. Neither is it acceptable nor should it be expected that Black women *must* straighten their hair in order to obtain or maintain employment! Such an expectation is clear grounds for a discrimination law suit. We must stop letting others dictate what is acceptable or unacceptable when it comes to wearing our natural hair. You will find that if you wear your natural hair with dignity and pride, in spite of the comments you may receive, in the long run, you will gain the respect of your co-workers, and others may overcome any inhibitions they may have toward wearing their natural hair. In fact, most women who do go natural are pleasantly surprised at the abundance of favorable comments they receive from coworkers and colleagues.

Incidentally, former talk show host Bertice Berry wore her hair locked on her nationally syndicated program in the early 1990s. It is our understanding that she was one of the first if not the first African American woman to wear locks on a daily show for the entire world to see! She was an excellent role model for any sister who contemplated wearing this particular natural style, but hesitated because they did not want to be the only one. Since that time, many women wear natural hairstyles in various popular media. Some still, however, straighten their hair or wear straight wigs and weaves in order to be accepted by White audiences.

Natural Hair: The Rebirth

The mid 1960s to the early 1970s was a period of cultural pride for many African Americans. Most African Americans chanted the words "Black is beautiful," and soul singer, James Brown, made the words, "Say it loud, I'm black and I'm proud," a national anthem for us. We wore "afros." Some wore short "fros" and some wore big "fros." Both men and women proudly wore dashikis and other African garb and jewelry. Unfortunately, this era did not last. As a people, we began to assimilate into Eurocentric ways of dressing and styling our hair with renewed energy. Shortly after this period James Brown who created the anthem I'm Black And I'm Proud, ultimately abandoned the afro and wore his hair in a relaxed style until his death in 2006.

In the 1980s the "jerri curl" became very popular in our community. This was a chemical process whereby the "natural curl" was replaced by a more loose, straight curl. Braiding and using extensions became popular toward the late 1980s. Many women, however, would relax their hair first before using extensions. Braids continue to be popular, and more women are wearing them minus the extensions.

The late 1980s to the present has seen the emergence of another hairstyle called the "wrap." This is a chemical process where the hair becomes "poker straight" and could be worn (short or long) in various straight hairstyles. A new trend began to develop in the mid to late 1990s. There was a gradual resurgence of women wearing their hair natural! Many women started opting, for various reasons, to shun chemical relaxers and hair pressing and are wearing their hair free of any straightening whatsoever!! These women appear in almost every age category and income bracket. The most common natural styles seen are short, symmetrically cut hairstyles, African locks, and twists. Some women also began braiding their hair without using extensions or relaxers.

There is, however, a difference between the cultural period of the 1960s and 1970s and the subsequent "awakening." Many of today's women and men are operating from an Afrocentric perspective.[2] More specifically, there is a "new consciousness" to go along with the natural hairstyles, one we think is more clearly defined than the one during the 1960s. These women (and men) are walking, talking, and thinking strictly from an African-centered perspective. There is a strong, unabashed identification with the rich, ancient history, practices, spirituality, and customs of Africa. For some, however, this new surge of natural hair wearing is just a passing fad. This is true particularly among adolescents. Nevertheless, it is one of the first steps towards the acknowledgment and acceptance of one's own cultural heritage and identity. We must start somewhere, and what better way to start than with our crowning glory?

Nekhena Evans states in her 1993 book, *Everything You Need To Know About Hairlocking*, that the five years prior to publishing her book there was a phenomenal rise in the number of African Americans wearing locks instead of a decline.[3] Since then there has been a semi-explosion of women wearing locks. For most of the late 1990s, it was more popular with men but because of our desire to emulate Whites (consciously or subconsciously), Black people have generally (since enslavement and colonialism) been ignorant about the care and maintenance of natural African hair. Due to the sudden rise of Black people wearing natural hair, salons that specialize in natural hair care started popping up all over the country. We correctly predicted in the first edition of this book that there would be an increase of these salons. In fact, in that edition (1996), we included a list of natural hair salons in the United States at the time which totaled forty-two salons. When we published the second version of the book in 2005, the number was well over five hundred that we could identify world wide within a thirty minute search of the internet. Since then and with the publication of this edition, the number of salons that cater to natural hair in various forms number in the thousands!

Additionally, with the advent of Youtube and other video-sharing websites, there are hundreds of videos available showing women and men how to care for their natural hair in whatever style they may choose. These developments have taken away previous excuses of ignorance about how to manage our hair. These developments have also set us on the course of reaching critical mass; that point where any movement or venture reaches the point where it will succeed despite the forces arrayed against it. In other words, when enough people start wearing natural hair, it will become the norm and to do otherwise would be seen as abnormal.

Some years ago New York State passed a bill that required licensing for the care of natural hair. The fact that natural African hair was even recognized to this extent was a major breakthrough. The passing of this law has undoubtedly helped revolutionize the black hair care industry and our attitudes toward it.

Many products are being sold on the market to aid Black people in grooming their natural hair. Numerous alternative products are now available to women who have used chemical straighteners and have had bad experiences with them. Some have had their hair literally fall out from the use of chemicals, never to grow back again, while others have, in some cases, received horrific burns to the scalp and skin due to the improper use of these chemicals.

Could it be that Black women are finally beginning to see the light? Unfortunately, most do not. However, some get it and more are waking up. One such case is former 1990s talk show host, Bertice Berry, who was interviewed after her shows success by Sophisticate's Black Hair, a hair magazine for Black women. When asked why she chose to wear her hair in the "natural" locked style, she replied,

It wasn't a choice. It is the way my hair grows. Why should I choose to perm my hair? It's natural and glorious, and I got tired of combing it! It made sense. [4]

If more black women thought as Ms. Berry does, there would be no need to write this book or one like it!

Credit should also be given to the Rastafarians. This religious group of Jamaicans has continued to maintain the tradition of hair-locking that originated in Africa. We must thank them for keeping this hairstyle more visible than it otherwise would have been. Ultimately, it is our vision that the majority of women of African descent will come to realize the outward beauty they possess, and will begin to wear their hair in whatever natural style they choose.

Opinion Poll: Black Women Wear *Natural* Hairstyles Because...

We surveyed an equal number of Black women who wear their hair in various *natural* hairstyles. Again, as in the previous survey, these women transcended all age groups and educational backgrounds. The participants were asked to check one or more reasons why they wear their hair natural. They were also asked to rate their reasons in order of importance.

An overwhelming 80% responded that the reason they wore their hair natural was because their natural hair was easier to manage. Only 25% of that number, however, listed this as their most important reason. A whopping 95% of the participants responded that they wore their hair natural because "it is an expression of my personal pride and cultural heritage." Over half, 53% of those participants, listed this as their number one reason. This evidence supports our earlier claim that many Black women are becoming more African conscious and appreciative of their God-given features.

75% of the participants responded that they did not want to use chemicals in their hair. A small percentage, just 10%, listed this as the number one reason for wearing their hair natural. 60% of the respondents felt that natural hair looked better, while only 10% of that group listed that as their number one reason.

33% of the participants said that their spouse/ boyfriend preferred them wearing their hair natural, however, none of the participants listed this as their number one reason for wearing natural hair. 20% of the participants responded that they wore their hair natural because it was different, and they liked to do different things with their hair. None of these participants listed that as their number one reason. A few comments given by some of these women were:

✦ *"Natural hair feels good and makes me feel good about myself."*

✦ *"I choose to wear my hair in its natural state because of my ancestors, and as African Americans, we should practice Afrocentricity in culture, health, hygiene, and philosophy."*

✦ *"It's a good, spiritual feeling to wear my hair like this."* *"Natural hair has given me something to call my own and to be proud of. This is my crown!"*

✦ *"I look good with it very short. I like it for the convenience."*

We also asked the women who wear natural hair if they planned to straighten their hair again. 80% of the participants responded "no", and 20% were undecided. None of the participants responded "yes."

It is apparent from the results of this poll that African women who choose, for whatever reason to wear natural hair, are beginning to realize the advantages as well as the "good feeling" they can have about themselves when choosing to wear their hair natural. The majority of the participants were proud to exhibit their natural "crowning glory."

Interestingly, a vast majority of these women also said that natural hair was easier to manage. Recall that in the first poll the majority of women responded that they straightened their hair *because it was easier to manage.* We ask, "Easier to manage than what?" Most Black women who wear their hair natural **NEVER STRAIGHTEN THEIR HAIR AGAIN.** When they make that "big switch" (and it is a big one for most of them), they are so turned on by the ease and manageability of caring for their natural hair, that they have told us they would never go back to the time and money spent in trying to maintain artificially straightened hair. As mentioned earlier, this has been made possible largely due to the emerging information we now possess regarding the general care and maintenance of our natural hair.

Perhaps, the biggest relief in wearing our hair natural is being able to walk out in the rain and not be afraid that it will "go back." Additionally, many Black women will not exercise because they are paranoid of perspiring around the hairline while others will not swim for fear of getting their hair wet. As one can see, wearing our hair natural eliminates most of these hang-ups and inconveniences. It also demonstrates that artificially straightened hair is not as easy to live with as some may think. Those who do straighten their hair are hardly ever satisfied with it. They inevitably become preoccupied with their hair "going back." They complain about it being too short and in some cases too long and unmanageable. They are on a perpetual treadmill of trying the latest fashion only to become disenchanted with it within six months or less.

One can never be satisfied trying to be like someone else. It may bring fleeting satisfaction, but in the long run it ends in frustration. Again, wearing natural hair eliminates these "bad hair days."

To all Nubian sisters, we say, don't knock it until you've tried it! LIBERATE YOUR HAIR! Remove yourself from the Eurocentric way of thinking that "straight" hair is the best hair. Stop making excuses for not wanting to be your true self inside and outside. The first step to loving each other is to really love OURSELVES!

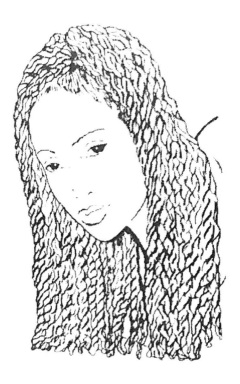

. . .there are more beauty shops in today's Black community than educational, cultural, economic or political institutions. Mass media has made it explicitly clear that the ideal is the 'European natural' and that the Germanic blond is the essence of 'correctness.' And we in our search for meaning generally go the way of European-American 'Correctness' not realizing that what is 'normal' for others may be deadly for us.
— Haki Madhubuti —

We feed a disease killing us.
— Ayi Kwei Armah —

Chapter 5

Your Health and Your Hair

When it comes to a discussion of African women's hair, no other area is more ubiquitously overlooked than health considerations. What are the implications of hair relaxers on one's health? What impact do the chemicals used to straighten hair have on the health of those who receive the application of the chemicals and those hair stylists who apply the chemicals?

The average and not so average person who receives a relaxer using harsh chemicals is totally unaware of the impact the chemicals have on the welfare of their health. Seldom, if ever, have they read a book or engaged in a serious discussion of how the chemicals used to relax their hair affects their body. This is true regardless of the educational background or socio-economic status. Most are equally uninformed on this subject to which they religiously subject themselves every few weeks. Yet, they allow these chemicals to be applied to their hair and scalp month after month and year after year. In addition, they have rarely, if ever, had a conversation with their doctor or hair stylist regarding the impact the chemicals have on their health.

Warning: Hair Chemicals Can Be Deadly To Your Health

Cosmetologist, Johnnie M. Miles, informs us of the following:

> *The damage from chemical[s] in most cases is so severe that hair can only be re-paired never revised. There seems to be serious damage to the hair follicle. The new growth is very weak, dry, breaks easily, has little or no natural oils... the hair becomes like straw.* [1]

Dermatologist, Stephen Mandy, observes,

> *I am seeing allergic reactions like weep blistered scalps and chemical burns from permanent wave solutions. That stuff (perm solution) is strong enough to break the chemical bonds of the hair; just imagine what it can do to your skin.* [2]

We accept, without question, that when a substance such as alcohol, liniment, sports cream, Ben-gay, etc. is applied to the skin to relieve muscle soreness or muscle spasms, it does not lie dormant on the epidermis (outer skin) but penetrates the other layers of skin entering the blood stream ultimately reaching the sore spot and providing relief. In this process, the ointment enters the blood stream enabling it to work more efficiently. In like manner, when chemicals, harsh or mild, are applied to the hair to straighten it, they come in contact with the scalp and penetrate the layers of skin there. They also enter into the blood stream, but their impact on the body is virtually unknown; at least it is not a popular item of discussion.

Medical doctor, Don Colbert, author of the book, *What You Don't Know May Be Killing You*, informs us that:

> *Your skin—even the skin on your scalp—is an organ that is able to absorb chemicals. What you put on your skin will end up in your body. If you don't believe me, try rubbing raw garlic on the bottom of your foot. Within minutes you will taste it in your mouth...Be sure you know what you are putting on your body's largest organ.* [3]

The good doctor goes on to say that,

> *Without your knowledge, poisons and cancer-causing substances can be absorbed slowly over time through your skin and lungs, and they can accumulate in your body...You can eat right, exercise, take supplements and do everything you know to live healthy and still be filling your body and the bodies of your loved ones with dangerous poisons. What you don't know about the products you use may be killing you and your family.* [4]

When we compare the effect of a solution (good or bad) that is placed on the skin with chemical solutions placed on the hair and scalp, the results are the same. In other words, if a chemical solution (harsh or mild) is powerful enough to straighten the natural coil of strong African hair for weeks, does it not also follow that those same chemicals would have some adverse or potentially dangerous effect on the body as well? This is even more compelling when we keep in mind that alcohol, Ben-gay and other such solutions are applied without the use of gloves to protect the hands, while the harsh and mild chemicals that are applied to the hair and scalp require the wearing of protective gloves to protect the hands of the stylist from burns. This is clear indication to any thinking person that this is a very dangerous, harmful and deadly activity.

What about the person receiving this treatment of chemicals, what protection do they have? The fact that the question has to be raised reveals the potential danger. The protection they receive is called a base, usually Vaseline. This base is applied around the edges of the hairline, the neck, and the ears to prevent burns. It is also supposed to be applied to the entire scalp, but rarely does this happen. In some cases, the hair is parted into sections where the base is applied to the scalp but usually not to the entire scalp.[5]

Even if it is applied to the entire scalp, some burning still occurs because only a thin coat of base may be applied since too much base would interfere with the ability of the chemical to straighten the hair. If the base is as protective as is claimed, why doesn't the stylist simply apply it with her/his uncovered hands instead of using gloves? Most, if not all stylists, would refuse such a suggestion on the grounds that it would be too messy, and that it goes against their cosmetological training. In addition, if they incurred severe burns they would have no legal recourse to claim damages.

That the base is not as protective as is claimed may be attested to by the burning that inevitably occurs before it is washed out. Most people who relax their hair have been conditioned to expect and accept the burning as a "natural" part of the process. Again, all this reveals the danger involved and the extent to which some people will go to alter or eliminate their African hair.

Hair Relaxers and Fibroids In Black Women

Medical research and studies show that Black women in the United States have 2-3 times more incidences of fibroids than white women. The research has been conducted for several decades investigating the issue trying to understand why the racial disparity exists. It was discovered that hair relaxers is one of the significant culprits or causes in Black women. In other words, the research showed a direct connection to high rates of fibroids and the use of relaxers in Black women.

The study was conducted in the late 1990's and early 2000's known as The Black Women's Health Study. The study made the following conclusion on the matter:

> ...the link between hair relaxers and increased fibroid risk is a significant discovery, both because it could partially explain the racial bias of uterine fibroids and because it serves as actionable information that enables women to moderate their exposure to the toxins that could contribute to the growth of fibroids. With this knowledge, women can make an informed decision about whether the potential cost of hair straightening treatments simply outweighs the beauty benefits.[6]

The Dangerous Ingredient in Hair Relaxers

Most people would be shocked to learn what is actually applied to the natural hair to make it straight and why it causes such an intense burning pain. Although there are many chemicals associated with relaxing the hair, the basic ingredient in relaxers or hair-straighteners is *sodium hydroxide* commonly known as lye.[7] *This chemical is extremely caustic, which means that it burns and damages the flesh on contact.* Caustic means that it burns and is corrosive which means that it gradually destroys or weakens something. The following is a typical warning found on relaxers containing sodium hydroxide or lye:

> **WARNING:** *This product contains Sodium Hydroxide (lye). Keep out of reach of children. Follow directions carefully to avoid skin and scalp burns, hair loss and eye injury…DO NOT USE if hair has been previously treated (i.e. blown dry, hot picked, braided, pressed and curled, relaxed, curly permed or any other treatment that would alter the natural curl formation)…if hair loss occurs, consult a physician.* (Authors' emphasis)

According to the Agency for Toxic Substances & Disease Registry (ATSDR), sodium hydroxide or lye, *"is very CORROSIVE and can cause severe burns in all tissues that it comes in contact with. Sodium hydroxide poses a particular threat to the eyes, since it can hydrolyze protein, leading to severe eye damage…or in extreme cases, blindness.*[8]

Lye is used as an industrial chemical and is found in some home cleaning solutions. Perhaps one of its best know uses is found in drain cleaners and oven cleaners and it is also used to make some soaps. It does not take much thought to understand that this is an extremely powerful and dangerous chemical. In fact, in the film *400 Years Without a Comb: The Inferior Seed*, it is shown that lye solutions used as a cleaner during our enslavement was accidentally discovered to straighten African hair when slave owners would force the heads of those enslaved into buckets of this solution as a form of punishment. The punishment caused severe burns to the skin, but surprisingly, it also made the hair of the African straight. This concoction was later modified and used by some enslaved males to straighten their hair in order to look more like their White slave-masters.[9]

What we see occurring today in beauty salons and manifested on the heads of the majority of Black women and some Black men in the United States, the Caribbean Islands, South America, and on the continent of Africa is a modification of this same process and a continuation of the same rationale as the first Africans who straightened their hair. Those other Africans who saw this initial attempt to straighten the African hair knew, without the benefit of "education," that the person doing it was attempting to be more like Whites. They also knew that this was an attempt to cover-up, hide, eliminate, or disguise their true African features and identity. It was no secret what was intended, but with the passage of time, modification of technique, the continued bombardment of White beauty standards as normal and accepted, and with the unabated attack and denigration of African beauty, it soon became an accepted practice to see more and more Africans, especially women, straightening their hair.

While it is important to note that the techniques might have changed, the rationale really remains the same. The practitioners, however, have intensified in their insistence that it is not an attempt to imitate White standards of beauty.

Needless to say, their rationale, to any thinking person, is transparent and superficial. Most are totally unaware of the historical origins that gave rise to this practice and the looming danger involved.

A Little Secret About No-Lye Relaxers

There are many products for straightening hair on the market called No-Lye relaxers. In our consultations with beauticians, we have repeatedly been informed that there really is no such thing as a No-Lye relaxer. These beauticians indicated to us that what is meant by No-Lye is that the amount of lye has been reduced in that product, but that they usually do contain some lye or a derivative. The fact that hair product companies have attempted to create such a product or the image of such a product is indicative of the health risks involved in straightening the hair. It is interesting to note that upon examination, one finds almost verbatim, the same warning on No-Lye relaxers as that found on relaxers that do not make this claim. The following instructions found on no-lye relaxer products makes the point:

> *This product contains no lye. Like any relaxer, however, it must be used carefully and in accordance with directions to avoid skin and scalp burns, hair loss and eye injury.* (Authors' emphasis)

The fact is there is no safe way to straighten one's hair using chemicals. Trained cosmetologist turned natural stylist,

Johnnie M. Miles states the following with regard to this point:

I am learned in the field, I have studied, read widely, listened to commercials, etc. And to this date have not found any perfectly safe chemical hair straightener. [10]

Speaking of the adverse affects of chemicals on Black women who straighten their hair, she notes:

The introduction of chemicals has brought with it balding, sore scalps, chemical burns, eye infections, total loss of hair immediately after perming, skin problems, headaches, etc. Many black women have become permanent wig wearers because of permanent loss of hair. [11]

Nightmare On Your Head and Other Horror Stories

Many of us are able to recall stories of "someone" whose hair may have fallen out because the chemicals were not "properly" applied; horror stories of severe burns received to the scalp and face, and/or allergic reactions that have been detrimental. A natural hairstylist and part owner of a natural hair salon recounted to us a personal horror story involving a relative who received a relaxer that caused such an adverse reaction that she was forced to miss nearly three weeks from work recuperating. Of course, she has finally decided to wear her hair natural, which is much safer. She also recounted another incident where a gentleman was blinded for a few days after some of the ingredients of a texturizer fell into his eyes.

Another story involves a friend of the authors that had more permanent results. This friend had a relaxer applied as usual, but on this occasion her hair washed down the drain during the rinse. This left her with patches of hair, which never grew back. In order to hide this unsightly appearance, she has been wearing wigs and scarves for more than thirty years! *We repeat, her hair never grew back...* She did not get a second chance.

This is not an isolated story, for there are untold numbers of Black women who are in this type of predicament or a similar one. Some have been more fortunate than others, but they keep taking the chances thinking it will never happen to them. Is it really worth the risk? It appears that millions of Black women think so since they would rather risk permanent baldness, patchy scalps or other unknown injury than wear their God-given natural hair.

The horror stories are endless and are a dime a dozen in the Black community. What is interesting is how such knowledge of the danger involved does not cause most of the victims to change their behavior. They usually attribute their misfortune to the stylist's lack of skill while they go in search of another stylist using the same chemicals that they believe will do a better job — this time. The search usually ends in disappointment and more frustration.

There are many people who never or rarely incur immediate adverse reactions from having relaxers put in their hair. The damage done, however, may be more insidious and in the long run just as harmful as immediate adverse reactions. Some Black women who use chemical straighteners throughout their lives will experience thinning around the hairline and at worst, will develop a receding hairline. Many of these women accept and justify this condition by claiming it is hereditary since their mother, aunts, and sisters may have the same condition. They usually do not recognize that what is really at work is that the other women in their family also straighten their hair. The condition may have more to do with straightening the hair and little or nothing to do with heredity.

A few years ago, a product, which claimed to be natural and danger-free for straightening the hair, received extensive television coverage. Black women were joyfully buying this product by the thousands because they thought they had found *the* answer to all their hair troubles. This appeared to be the case until many of them experienced unhealthy reactions to this product. As we understand it, some of them have sued the makers of this product and the product is no longer available.

Like it or not the bottom line is this; prolonged application of any chemical, especially those used in hair relaxers, to such an important and delicate part of the body as the head is bound to have some disastrous consequences.

Even if there existed such a product that was all-natural and did not jeopardize one's health, the core issue and concern would remain—**why the desire to straighten the hair in the first place?** *The method used to* *straighten the hair is really inconsequential, but the motivation, the rationale; the logic for doing it is paramount and may adversely affect both your physical and your mental health.*

Conquering The Fear of Natural Hair

What we have said is the truth. Regardless of whether you currently wear your hair natural or straight, the truth of what we have said can easily be tested. You need but look at your relatives, your friends, your acquaintances, and maybe even yourself. They have accepted straightening hair as correct and normal. Despite the hard-core truth of our observations and experiences, many will still attempt to deny truth and continue to straighten their hair however faulty their justification. Why? It's primarily due to fear.

Fear cripples your actions, sometimes even in the light of truth. It prevents you from doing what you *know* is right; from realizing your full potential; from accepting the truth. Although it is a sad but true fact, fear of being fully Black prevents most Black women from wearing their hair natural. Fear of what they will look like with their natural hair; fear of what others will say to their face and behind their backs; fear of rejection; fear of what whites, Asians, and others will think and say. It is fear that does all this—nothing more nothing less. It is fear—not freedom of choice, or ease of manageability, or unemployment that prevents them from going natural.

This fear may be likened to a monster that has been created out of their imagination. They believe that it will grab them and eat them alive if they should go natural. Like most creations of the mind, it is believed and accepted to be true. In order to conquer this fear or any fear, you must first accept the truth. Acceptance of the truth will liberate you from the monster of your mind.

We know of no one who has gone natural that has been eaten up by any monsters. They work in all areas of life as teachers, politicians, lawyers, actors and actresses, astronauts, judges, musicians, journalists, clerks, computer specialists, talk show hosts, writers, entrepreneurs, salespeople, mail carriers, principals, administrators, managers, ministers, engineers, college presidents, etc. Again, we know of no one who has been eaten up by monsters when they went "natural." Yes, it does take courage to go natural. Those who do wear their hair natural will tell you that it is an act of courage for them to make that move. In making that move, however, they will also tell you that they have been liberated. They are beautiful, they have a variety of choices, they have no problems managing their hair, and they are employed.

What monster do you fear will grab you and eat you up if you go natural? Are you afraid of the natural hair monster? Remember that it is in your mind not in reality. You and those around you have created this illusion. But you have the power to kill the monster and be liberated from your self-imposed exile of shame.

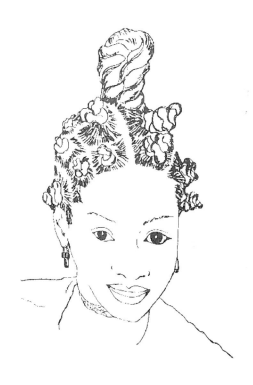

UJAMAA (Cooperative Economics) To build and maintain our own stores, shops and other businesses and to profit from them together.
—Fourth Principle of the Nguzo Saba for Kwanzaa —

Chapter 6

Your Money and Your Hair

The amount of money spent by our community for hair products and services is astronomical. The hair care products industry rakes in over $1 billion dollars annually, while the hair care industry exceeds $500 million dollars annually.[1] Casual observation would inform us that this is very big business, but African participation in it as manufacturers and retailers is quickly vanishing. This is because white-owned and Asian-owned companies have moved into the business of Black hair and they are reaping overwhelming profits, while Black-owned businesses are closing shop.

There are a few reasons for this according to a recent Newsweek article. The article first points out that due to slow growth, white-owned companies have calculatingly and deliberately targeted Blacks. Secondly, the article asserts that Blacks tend to spend more than Whites on hair care and hair care products. We add another factor to this equation; Blacks, as a group, do not vigilantly and diligently spend their dollars with black-owned companies. This is true even though a survey conducted by the Chicago based research firm, Viewpoint, Inc., revealed that 79% of African

Americans would spend their dollars with black-owned brands if they in fact knew which ones were black-owned.

The Money Trail: From Your Pocket to... *"Their"* Bank Account

Many times we are fooled by the name of a product into thinking that Blacks own the company. Dark & Lovely, African Pride, and Right on Curl are a few examples of white-owned companies marketing Black hair products using catch phrases from our culture and heritage. For example, African Pride products use the colors Red, Black, and Green on all of their products, and, of course, the name *African* would lead one to think it is an African-owned company. In fact, a few years ago the White owners of African Pride, Shark Products of Brooklyn, New York, attempted to sue B & J Sales Company, an Atlanta based African American hair product company, for using the name "African" on its products![2] Many of us naively think white-owned companies would never do anything like that, but because of our naiveté, as noted in Newsweek, "*White businesses now control 50 percent of the ethnic* [Black] *hair-care market—and they'll elbow out more black (sic) businesses if, as expected, Procter & Gamble, Gillette and Chanel (sic) enter the industry.*"[3]

The arrogance of some of the white-owned companies may be better understood in light of the following statement made by Revlon's Professional Products Division president, Irving J. Bottner, who predicted:

The black-owned businesses will disappear. They'll all be sold to the white companies...black consumers buy quality products...their black brothers didn't do them any good. [4]

In response to this gratuitous statement, *Essence* magazine followed up by announcing "it would no longer accept advertising from Revlon Inc., an account worth $400,000 in revenues last year." [5] In the same article, it was correctly noted that Revlon [and other white-owned companies] imitates almost everything created by Black companies. Bottner's statement also inferred that Black companies do not make good products, which is absolutely untrue. Most of the products sold by black-owned companies are tantamount to or better than those produced by white-owned companies.

At the retail level, it is appalling whose stores are situated in Black communities selling products to groom the hair of Black folks. But what epitomizes our own lack of diligence is the way we as a community mindlessly patronize these stores; stores that cater to approximately 95% Black consumers, but rarely do these retailers employ Black job seekers. What adds insult to injury is that black-owned retail stores in the same city/town, which provide job opportunities for themselves and other Blacks are not patronized by the Black community. We are not suggesting that these retailers are the answer to all Black unemployment woes, but they do provide invaluable opportunities and experience for many Black people and could probably provide even more if they were adequately patronized.

We are also aware that in some cases these Black retailers may not provide the type of service they should or they may not stock the particular product that one may want. Instead of abandoning these retailers and going to those outside our community, we offer the following suggestions:

1. *If you are not treated with courteous and skilled service, approach the owner/manager in a friendly manner and inform her/him that you make it a point to patronize their business, but that you are disappointed with the service you have received.*

2. *If the store does not carry the product you are seeking or if they are out of it, ask them in a friendly manner if they would be able to order it for you or when and if they will have it in stock again.*

We stress that the owner/manager be approached in a friendly and courteous manner emphasizing your intention to patronize their business. This approach will help the store improve its service and product line. Most owners welcome such criticisms and suggestions because they are intent on serving the community and realizing a profit. This approach also keeps them accountable for the type of service they provide and does not allow them to treat customers in any fashion. It may be that they have not been taught the finer nuances of running a business, and those of us who know how it should be done might help them to succeed by taking an active interest. If, on the other hand, you, the consumer, leave the store unsatisfied intending never to return, you will, in all likelihood, tell your relatives and friends which may influence them to not patronize this hair product retailer. In such cases, it may not be long before a GOING OUT OF BUSINESS sign is posted—then we all lose.

The point to understand in all of this is that Black consumers and Black businesses must be conscious and deliberate in their dealings with each other. The consumer must exercise their responsibility to patronize the business and point out its weaknesses and strengths. The retailer must be willing to take constructive criticism from those "nonprofessionals" and make needed improvements. These points and this discussion go beyond the hair products store and may be applied equally to any business in our community.

Snakes In The Grass

Realizing that many African American consumers are not aware of the tactics used by white-owned companies to capture their dollars by using names suggesting African culture or by using graphics that serve the same purpose, we have provided a list of white-owned companies and brands which many believe are black-owned and a list of black-owned companies and brands. The lists include both hair and cosmetic products.

Although we have attempted to be as thorough as possible, this is not an exhaustive list. Consumers should keep in mind that buy-outs do occur wherein a black-owned company may be purchased by a white-owned company operating under the former product labeling. Such is the case with Johnson Products Company, which was formerly a black-owned company that was sold to the Ivax Company.

This company is not to be confused with Johnson Publishing Company, which, as we understand it, is still black-owned. Some of the products in our list may be Johnson products. Thus, consumers must look carefully at all hair care products before buying if they wish to support black-owned companies.

Regarding these lists, we are not endorsing any particular product, and we do not concur with many of the products manufactured and marketed by some of the black-owned companies. Obviously, many of them are in the business of marketing products used to straighten hair. We have provided the lists to educate and inform consumers so that they may be better able to make intelligent decisions. The bulk of these companies and products listed were obtained from a study conducted by ViewPoint, Inc., a Chicago-based market research firm. We added those not included in their research through direct contact with the manufacturers or the owners of the product. Although we have confidence in the study conducted by ViewPoint, Inc., we recommend that consumers double check to insure their accuracy.

The businesses that thrive and flourish in our communities have been a reflection of our choices to support them as a community. Since they realize larger profits, they usually have the wherewithal for more media advertisement. This provides them with even larger profits. When we rearrange our thinking, it will be reflected in our buying habits. We must support those businesses that support both our community and us, and perhaps we will then begin to realize a degree of economic and cultural empowerment and liberation.

AFRICAN AMERICAN OWNED BRANDS & COMPANIES

Actramoist
African Natural
Afrikan Republic
African Royale
African Wonders
Afroveda
American Pleasure
Ashaway (Lotion)
Asholine (Body Creme)
Ausome
Baby Love
Black magic (for men)
Bodi
Bonner Bros (BB)
Boundless tresses
California Curl
Carefree Curl
Carol's Daughter
Classy Curl
Claudio St. James
Design Essentials
Designer Touch
Diva by Cindy
Don't B Bald
Donnie's
Dudley
Duke(*Owned by Johnson Publishing Co.*)
Ebone Cosmetics(*Owned by Johnson Publishing Co.*)
Elentee
Essations Multi-textural
Ethnic Gold Cosmetics
Exrasi Hair Products
Everlasting

Fashion Fair (Owned by Johnson Publishing Co.)
Gentille Products
Global Beauty
Hairveda
flora L'original Hair Products
Isoplus
Just For Me
Kizure
Light 'N Free
Locks of Luster
Luster Products
Mizani Oh So Soft
Mr. Leonardo Hair Products
Natural Oasis
Nature's Image
Oil of K
Oran's International
Oyin Products
PCJ
Perm Repair
Phase 2
Pink Oil
Praises All Natural Beauty Products
Princess Kayla's Natty Locks
Prosonique
Razac
Raven(*Owned by Johnson Publishing Co.*)
Relaxed Look
Royal Roots
S-Curl
Simply Satin Cosmetics
Sizta 2 Sizta
Soft & Beautiful

Sportin Waves
Stone Fox Panty Hose
Tender Care
The Wrappe
Upturn

Vitale
Wave by Design
Wave Nouveau
Wonder Gro Hair Products
Worlds of Curls

WHITE OWNED BRANDS & COMPANIES

African Pride
African Best
African Gold
Affirm
Afro Sheen
Always Natural
Ambi Skin Cremes
Artra Skin Cream
Bantu
Black Opal
Bone Strait
Brown Sugar and Afro-Tique Stocking/Panty Hose
Bump Fighter
Care Free
Clairol
Creme of Nature
Dark & Lovely
Dark & Natural
Dax
Doo Gro (Korean Revlon)
Dr. Miracles
Fabulaxer (Korean Revlon)
Flori Roberts Cosmetics
Gentle Treatment (Johnson & Johnson)
IC Products (Fantasia; Korean)
Infusium 23
LeKair Products
Let's Jam (L'oreal)
Long Aid
Lustrasilk *(Not Luster Products which is Black -owned)*
Magic Shave
Mane N'Tall
Mizani (Korean Revlon)
Motions (Alberts Culver)
Murray's Hair Pomade
Nadinola

New Era
Nexus
No Blade Shave
Palmer's Cocoa Butter Lotion and Creme
Perm Repair
Pernevu
Posner's Easy Wave and Mink Pro
Queen Helene Rebound
Relax and Natural
Revlon Right on Curl
Royal Crown
Sebastian
Shades of You Cosmetics (Maybelline)
Skin Success
Sof N-Free
Soft and Beautiful
Smooth n Shine
Sta-Sof-Fro
Sulfur 8
Takedown Hair
TCB
The Dream of X
Ultra Sheen
Ultra Star
Vitale
Waterless Shave
Wave Nouveau

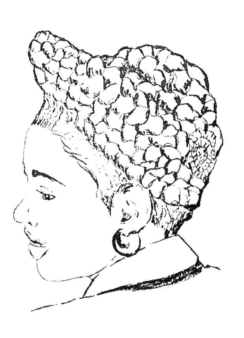

What I insist on is the poison must be eliminated once and for all.
　　　　　　　—Frantz Fanon —

Chapter 7

Looking In The Wrong Mirror

It matters if you are Black or White. In a society where only White people are portrayed as beautiful, good, kind, etc.; where Whites have the power: economical, political, social, educational, military and otherwise; where power is reserved for Whites only; where the image of the Creator and other heavenly entities are White only, in such a society, those who are not White, in attempting to garner to themselves the trappings of power, would endeavor to imitate those in power. Their attempts to receive that power, actual or assumed, means they must relinquish their ethnic or racial identity. Such a setup leads them to feel and think they must approximate Whites in appearance and attitude in order to have value and self-worth. In order to justify their imitation of white people's hair, they rationalize the irrational by appealing to such notions as ease of manageability, popular culture, freedom of choice, and current trends/fads; the epitome of conformity. It matters if you are Black or White.

In a society where Black people are portrayed relentlessly as ugly, bad, evil, etc.; where Blacks have no power economical, political, social, educational, military and otherwise, except as Whites allow it; where power for Blacks is reserved only for those who are more White than Black;

where the physical features of Blacks are denigrated and disdained and reinforced through books, magazines, newspapers, television, radio, movies, religion and educational institutions; where Blacks are denied their divine humanity; and where the image of the devil and evil is depicted and associated with being Black; and where no Blacks are part of the "heavenly" drama, in such a society those who are Black would not associate power and beauty with being Black. They would exhibit entrenched disdain for their features and contempt for those features in others like them. They would use negative and derogative terms in reference to their own physical features, while speaking always in laudatory and praiseworthy terms regarding White people's features. They would conclude that the less Black they are, the more divine, the more beautiful, the more powerful they will become. They would associate Black with evil, dirty, unworthy, and ugly in such a society. Moreover, they would teach their children these things.

In order to justify their denigration, disdain, and contempt for Black features, they would appeal to the axiom of being in Rome and doing as the Romans; they would assert that just because they hide, alter, deny, or cover-up their Black features is no indication of how Black they are or how devoted to Black causes they may be in their hearts. Such people tend to be shallow, false to themselves and others. But mostly they are ignorant of what has happened to them, how it was done, and how they unwittingly perpetuate it. There are too many of us in a deep state of denial when we believe or agree that people who straighten their hair are not attempting to imitate White people's hair. The historical record attests to this, and the society over centuries has repeatedly taught this lesson. White is beautiful in western society and Black, well Black appears to be only beautiful as long as it's acceptable.

This all speaks to the evidence of a continued enslaved mentality that we do not wish to acknowledge. The recent past has reshaped our perceptions of ourselves and of the world. In the more distant past we (Africans) shaped the world according to our standards, according to our perceptions and values. We valued one another in form and in symbol. If we are to survive and flourish, if we are to be victorious, we must revisit our distant past and reclaim and recapture that of which we were robbed. And what was it that was taken from us? We were robbed of our mind, the sense of our real identity, and what is valuable in us. We were robbed of our confidence in ourselves and true love of ourselves. This theft destroyed in us the idea of ourselves as humans. It sabotaged the idea of us as valuable and beautiful. It twisted our understanding of the fact that imitation is suicide, and that envy is ignorance. In such a mindset, and in such a framework, where we are hell-bent on straightening our hair, we are also, however ignorantly, hell-bent on the destruction of African hair.

In order to circumvent this destruction, it is incumbent upon parents and other adults to develop a sense of their personal value. They must realize that their value as humans does not reside in the illusion that the texture of one's hair determines value or the lack thereof. This message must be passed on to their children and all Black children. Our words must coincide with our actions. It is a contradiction in reality to tell Black children how beautiful they are while attempting to alter, hide, or disguise the very features that make the child beautiful. Children tend to imitate adults, and what we adults value is also what our children will value and emulate. Black folk's hair is beautiful!! There is nothing pertaining to our hair of which we should be ashamed or embarrassed. When we understand this, we will realize that we have been hiding the best kept secret, and in so finding, we may gain a greater degree of liberation. It is said that, "You shall know the truth and it shall set you free." Ase!

NOTES

Chapter 1

1. Calvin R. Robinson, Redman Battle, and Edward W. Robinson, Jr., *The Journey of the Songhai People*, 2nd ed., (Philadelphia: The Pan African Organization, 1987), 56.
2. Nekhena Evans, *Everything You Need to Know About Hairlocking: Dread, African & Nubian Locks* (New York: New Bein' Press, 1993), 16.
3. Ibid.
4. Consult Evans for a fuller discussion of the spiritual aspects of African hair.
5. Robinson, *Songhai*, 42-43.
6. Ibid., 43.
7. We are also aware that there was a mixture of Blacks with the indigenous populations in the Americas (so called Indians), which accounts for some of the straight hair of some Blacks.

Chapter 2

1. Na'im Akbar, *Chains and Images of Psychological Slavery* (Jersey City: New Mind Productions, 1984), 22.
2. Sonja Peterson-Lewis, "Aesthetic Practices Among African American Women," in *The African Aesthetic: Keeper of the Tradition*, ed. Kariamu Welsh-Asante, Contributions in the Afro-American and African Studies, no. 153 (Westport: Greenwood Press, 1993), 105.
3. Akbar, 21.
4. Peterson-Lewis, 106.
5. Ibid., 105.
6. Willie Morrow, *400 Years Without A Comb: The Inferior Seed* (San Diego, Calif.: California Curl, 1989), video.
7. Haki R. Madhubuti, *Enemies: The Clash of Races* (Chicago: Third World Press, 1978), ii.
8. Akbar, 22.

Chapter 3

1. "nappy." Merriam-Webster.com. 2019. https://www.merriam-webster.com/dictionary/nappy (5 August 2019)
2. Molefi Kete Asante, *Kemet, Afrocentricity, and Knowledge* (Trenton: Africa World Press, 1990), 11.

Chapter 4

1. There are number of good books on the market that deal with how to care for African/natural hair. We recommend the following:

> Lonnice Brittenum Bonner, *Good Hair: For Colored Girls Who've Considered Weaves When the Chemical Became Too Ruff* (New York: Crown Trade Paperbacks, 1990). This book describes how to make the transition from relaxers to natural styles.

> Nekhena Evans, *Everything You Need to Know About Hairlocking: Dread, African & Nubian Locks* (New York: New Bein' Press, 1993). For those curious about locks and those thinking about making that transition, this is an excellent book.

> Johnnie M. Miles, *Naturally Beautiful You: A Guide to the Care, History, and Culture of Black/African Hair* (Linden: Naturally Beautiful You Salon, 1985). The title speaks for itself. This is an excellent source also but unfortunately is out of print.

Additionally, there are numerous Youtube videos explaining how to manage and style natural hair.

2. Afrocentricity is a term coined by Dr. Molefi Kete Asante of Temple University, which means "literally placing African ideals at the center of any analysis that involves African culture and behavior." This book is an Afrocentric project. See his work *The Afrocentric Idea* (Philadelphia: Temple University

Press, 1987), 6. And *Afrocentricity*, rev. ed., (Trenton: Africa World Press, 1988), 6.

3. Nekhena Evans, *Everything You Need to Know About Hairlocking: Dread, African & Nubian Locks* (New York: New Bein' Press, 1993), xv.
4. *Sophisticate's Black Hair: Styles and Care Guide*, 1994.

Chapter 5

1. Johnnie M. Miles, *Naturally Beautiful You: A Guide to the Care, History and Culture of Black/African Hair* (Linden: Naturally Beautiful You Salon, 1985), 17.
2. Karyn Snead, *"Beautician's Chemicals Pose An Ugly Danger,"* Fort Lauderdale News & Sun Sentinel, 1986.
3. Don Colbert, MD, *What You Don't Know May Be Killing You* (Lake Mary: Siloam Press, 2000), 211.
4. Colbert, 206.
5. This is the assertion of beauticians we consulted.
6. "The Straight Truth: Hair Relaxers and Fibroids." (2019, August 6). Retrieved from https://acessaprocedure.com/2016/08/25/the-straight-truth-hair-relaxers-and-fibroids/
7. There are other chemicals used in relaxers and other hair products that pose health dangers. For example, methyl chloride (used in aerosol hair sprays). Studies conducted by the National Toxicology Program indicated that it causes malignant liver and lung tumors in lab animals, i.e., cancer. The FDA predicted that one out of every 100 beauty-workers exposed to this chemical will die of cancer.
8. "Toxic Substances Portal - Sodium Hydroxide." (2019, August 6) Retrieved from https://www.atsdr.cdc.gov/MMG/MMG.asp?id=246&tid=45
9. Willie Morrow, *400 Years Without A Comb: The Inferior Seed* (San Diego, Calif.: California Curl, 1989), video.
10. Miles, 16.
11. Ibid., 17.

Chapter 6

1. Penelope Wang and Maggie Malone, "Targeting Black Dollars: White-Owned Companies Muscle Minority Firms Out of the Hair-Care Market," *Newsweek*, (October 13, 1986), 54-55.
2. Lisa Jones, "Skin Trade: Africa™," *Village Voice*, August 18, 1993.
3. Wang, "Targeting Black Dollars," 54.
4. Christine Dugas and Kenneth Dreyfack, "A Gaffe at Revlon Has The Black Community Seething," *Business Week*, (February 9, 1987), 36-37.
5. Ibid.

Appendix (A)

QUESTIONNAIRE

Please check the following reasons **why you wear your hair in a natural style** *(i.e. short or long natural, locks, braids with unpermed hair)*. You may check more than one:

____A. My hair is easier to manage when it's in its natural state.
____B. My spouse/boyfriend prefers my hair natural.
____C. It's different, and I like to do different things with my hair.
____D. Natural hair looks better.
____E. Wearing my hair natural is an expression of my personal pride and cultural heritage.
____ F. I do not want to use any chemicals in my hair.
____ G. I have never given it any thought.
____ H. Other_____

If you checked more than one reason above, please use the space below to rate your reasons in order of importance to you:

_____

Do you plan to ever straighten your hair again?
Yes   ( )   No   ( )   Undecided   ( )

Please check the age category that applies to you:

(a)   14-20   ( )
(b)   21-30   ( )
(c)   31-40   ( )
(d)   41-50   ( )
(e)   over 50 ( )

Please check your educational level:

(a)   Did not complete high school   ( )
(b)   High School Diploma   ( )
(c)   Completed two years of college ( )
(d)   Completed four years of college ( )
(e)   Graduate degree   ( )
(f)   Post graduate degree   ( )

(g)   Other _____ ( )

Thank you for your cooperation in helping us complete this study.
(Used in poll Chapter 4)

Appendix (B)

QUESTIONNAIRE

Please check the following reasons **why you straighten your
hair** (i.e. hot comb or chemically). You may check more than one:

_____   A. My hair is easier to manage when it is straight.
_____   B. My spouse/boyfriend prefers my hair straight.
_____   C.It's the style. Mostly everyone else straightens their
hair.
_____   D. Straight hair looks better.
_____   E. My employer would look unfavorably at my wearing
my hair in a natural style.
_____   F. I feel that natural hair is unattractive.
_____   G. I have never given it any thought.
_____   H.
Other_____

If you checked more than one reason above, please use the
space below to rate your reasons in order of importance to you:

_____

Do you plan to ever straighten your hair again?

Yes   ( )   No   ( )   Undecided   ( )

Please check the age category that applies to you:

(a)   14-20   ( )
(b)   21-30   ( )
(c)   31-40   ( )
(d)   41-50   ( )
(e)   over 50 ( )

Please check your educational level:

(a) Did not complete high school   ( )
(b) High School Diploma   ( )
(c) Completed two years of college   ( )
(d) Completed four years of college   ( )
(e) Graduate degree   ( )
(f) Post graduate degree   ( )
(g) Other _____   ( )

Thank you for your cooperation in helping us complete this study.
(Used in poll Chapter 4)

Selected Bibliography

Akbar, Na'im. *Chains and Images of Psychological Slavery.* Jersey City: New Mind Productions, 1984.

Ani, Marimba. *Yurugu: An African-Centered Critique of European Cultural Thought and Behavior.* Trenton: Africa World Press, 1994.

Armah, Ayi Kwei. *Two Thousand Seasons.* Chicago: Third World Press, 1979.

Asante, Molefi K. *The Afrocentric Idea.* Philadelphia: Temple University Press, 1987.

_____ *Afrocentricity.* Rev. ed. Trenton: Africa World Press, 1988.

_____ *Kemet, Afrocentricity and Knowledge.* Trenton: Africa World Press, 1990.

Bonner, Lonnice Brittenum. *Good Hair: For Colored Girls Who've Considered Weaves When the Chemicals Became Too Ruff.* New York: Crown Trade Paperbacks, 1990.

Colbert, Don. *What You Don't Know May Be Killing You.* Lake Mary: Siloam Press, 2000.

Dugas, Christine and Dreyfack, Kenneth. "A Gaffe at Revlon Has the Black Community Seething." *Business Week* (Feb. 9, 1987), 36-37.

Evans, Nekhena. *Everything You Need to Know About Hairlocking: Dread, African & Nubian Locks.* New York: New-Bein' Press, 1993.

Fanon, Frantz. Black Skin, White Masks. New York: Grove Press, Inc., 1967.

Green, Kim. "The Pain of Living the Lye." *Essence* (June 1993), 38.

Haley, Alex. *The Autobiography of Malcolm X.* New York: Ballantine Books, 1965.

Jones, Kenneth M. "Say Brother." *Essence* (October 1985), 8.

Jones, Lisa. "Skin Trade: Africa™." *The Village Voice.* August 18, 1993.

McKinney, Gwen. "Being Me, Naturally." *Essence* (September 1985), 167.

Miles, Johnnie M. *Naturally Beautiful You: A Guide to the Care, History, and Culture of Black/African Hair.* New Jersey: Naturally Beautiful You Salon, 1985.

Peterson-Lewis, Sonja. "Aesthetic Practices Among African American Women" *The African Aesthetic: Keeper of the Traditions.* Edited by Kariamu Welsh-Asante. Westport: Greenwood Press, 1993.

Robinson, Edward, Battle, Redman, Robinson, Calvin. *The Journey of the Songhai People.* 2nd ed. Philadelphia: Pan African Federation Organization, 1987.

Sinclair, Abiola. "Black Hair and the Cultural/Political Movement" Part 1 *The New York Amsterdam News.* New York: February 6, 1993. p. 26.

Snead, Karyn. "Beautician's Chemicals Pose An Ugly Danger" *Fort Lauderdale News & Sun Sentinel*, 1986.

Wang, Penelope and Malone, Maggie. "Targeting Black Dollars: White-Owned Companies Muscle Minority Firms Out of the Hair-Care Market." *Newsweek* (Oct. 13, 1986), 54-55.

Weathers, Natalie. "The Hair Thing" *The Burning Torch.* Temple University vol. 2 no. 1, 1990.

Wilson, Judith. "Beauty Rites: Towards an Anatomy of Culture in Africa-American Women's Art." *International Review of African-American Art* (11:3, 1994), 11- 17, 47-55.

Index

Acknowledgments

There are so many to thank for helping make this project a success. First and foremost, we thank the Creator and the Ancestors for ultimately enabling us to complete and continue this work. This book was inspired by the work and encouragement of the late Redman Battle and Calvin Robinson who first broached this subject matter in a Pan African Federation Organization class taken by Kamau many years ago. We owe them an incalculable debt, and to them we say, Ase!

We thank our families, the late Arberdella and Joseph Graham and the late Marion and Thomas Green, for their support and encouragement. We are also grateful to the many friends who encouraged us to write a book on this subject. Among them we thank Tommy, Kenny, and Joseph Graham, Jr.

We also thank Professor Molefi K. Asante for his faith in us and for his encouragement. For their critiques, reviews, and suggestions, we are indebted to Pearl & Mark Christian, Audrey Davis, Gail Scott-Bey, Victor M. Vega, John Dunning, Sr., Leslie Carter, Johnnie Miles, Marvetta Troop, LaVerne Johnson, and Sharon Owens.

Thank you to my (Kamau) former students at Mercer County College and William Paterson University for your help and my current students at Northampton Community College. The technical aspects of some of the material would not have been possible without the expert advice of the late Lola Harps, Eisha Pitts, Alfrado Taylor, Troy Harrison, and Geneva Hall. Thanks to Sister Griots (Estina Baker and Akanke Nur) for their advice and encouragement.

We would like to thank our daughters Aliya and Ayanna for their steadfastness, encouragement and for being extraordinary examples of young women who have, thus far, worn natural hair their entire lives. We thank each other for the other's patience, intellect, and understanding of this topic!

Last but not least, a hearty thank you to all the women who gave of their time to participate in the surveys. Ase!

About The Authors

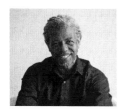

Kamau Kenyatta is a professor of African World Studies. He currently teaches at Northampton Community College in Bethlehem, PA. He is the owner of Kenyatta Digital Agency and is an in demand speaker for conferences, seminars and workshops.

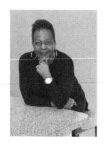

Janice Kenyatta is a retired Educator/ Administrator. She writes from personal experiences and from interaction through classroom instruction and seminars and is a sought after speaker for various events.

For speaking events such as:
- keynotes
- seminars
- panels
- workshop

Email the authors at speak@trueblackhair.com

Visit us at www.TrueBlackHair.com

For interviews, podcasts, and other media call 570-856-5178.